PINEAL
TUMORS

PINEAL

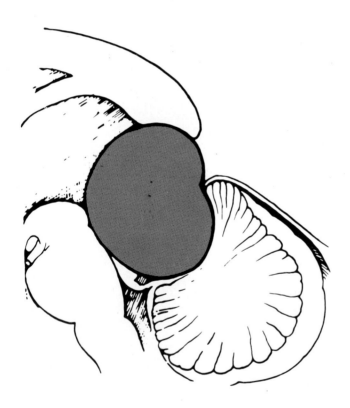

TUMORS

EDITED BY

Henry H. Schmidek, M.D., F.A.C.S.

PROFESSOR AND CHAIRMAN
DEPARTMENT OF NEUROSURGERY
HAHNEMANN MEDICAL COLLEGE AND HOSPITAL
PHILADELPHIA, PENNSYLVANIA

MASSON Publishing USA, Inc.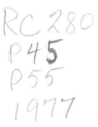
New York • Paris • Barcelona • Milan

ISBN 0-89352-007-1

Library of Congress Catalog Card Number: 77-78560

Printed in the United States of America

This book is dedicated
to my wife, Mary, and to my children,
Ian, Alexandra and Jared.

Foreword

CANCER MANAGEMENT

In 1977, the American Cancer Society estimates that about 690,000 people will be diagnosed as having cancer. These estimates of the incidence of cancer are based upon data from the National Cancer Institute's Third National Survey (1969–1971). About 230,000 or one-third of those in whom the diagnosis is established will be alive at least five years after treatment. About 115,000 of those who will die in 1977 might have been saved by earlier treatment.

The purpose of this series of monographs is to bring to the practicing physician, as rapidly as possible, the major strides being made in the diagnosis and treatment of cancer. A quiet revolution in cancer management is resulting from a combination of more appropriate and exact diagnostic techniques, the implementation of multidisciplinary, multimodal treatment techniques, the identification of factors influencing patient prognosis, and more appropriate and careful follow-up examinations and evaluations.

The series in *Cancer Management* will address the various problems inherent in diagnosis and treatment, with emphasis on new advances in those areas. Making such information available to the practicing physician in a coordinated, composite fashion will have a significant impact on earlier diagnosis, more appropriate treatment selection, and broader implementation of newer treatment information.

Luther W. Brady
Vincent T. De Vita, Jr.
June 1977

Contributors

Axelrod, Lloyd, M.D., Assistant Professor of Medicine, Harvard Medical School, Assistant in Medicine, Massachusetts General Hospital, Boston, Massachusetts

Brady, Luther, M.D., Professor and Chairman, Department of Radiation Therapy, Hahnemann Medical College and Hospital, Philadelphia, Pennsylvania

de Girolami, Umberto, M.D., Assistant Professor of Pathology (Neuropathology), University of Massachusetts Medical School, Worchester, Massachusetts

Gonzalez, Carlos, M.D., Associate Professor of Medicine, Head, Section of Neuroradiology, Hahnemann Medical College and Hospital, Philadelphia, Pennsylvania

Grossman, Charles B., M.D., Assistant Professor of Radiology, Head, Section of Neuroradiology, The Milton S. Hershey Medical Center, Pennsylvania State University College of Medicine, Hershey, Pennsylvania

Schmidek, Henry H., M.D., F.A.C.S., Professor and Chairman, Department of Neurosurgery, Hahnemann Medical College and Hospital, Philadelphia, Pennsylvania

Wray, Shirley H., M.D., F.R.C.P., Associate Professor of Neurology, Harvard Medical School, Associate Neurologist, Massachusetts General Hospital, Director of Neuro-Ophthalmology, Massachusetts Eye and Ear Infirmary, Boston, Massachusetts

Wurtman, Richard J., M.D., Professor of Endocrinology and Metabolism, Department of Nutrition and Food Science, Laboratory of Neuroendocrine Regulation, Massachusetts Institute of Technology, Cambridge, Massachusetts

Contents

Introduction

Two groups of investigators currently explore the pineal organ: neurosurgeons and their colleagues in related clinical disciplines, who record the natural history of pineal tumors and who treat people suffering from these neoplasms; and basic scientists, who study the role of the pineal in normal physiology as well as the pharmacologic effects of its constituents.

This long-needed and unique book will do much to assist clinicians. It provides them with a thorough description of the neoplasms that occur in the pineal region, from the perspectives of all of the various approaches utilized to study and to treat these tumors. By focussing attention on pineal tumors as a significant clinical problem, *Pineal Tumors* should also attract the interest of basic scientists and foster collaborative studies between this group of investigators and the physicians who have access to afflicted patients.

During the past 2 years, excellent methods have been developed for measuring levels of melatonin and other putative pineal hormones in blood, cerebrospinal fluid, and urine. In each of these body fluids, the levels of melatonin have been shown to vary with parallel daily rhythms. These chemical approaches have yet to be applied to the study of pineal tumors or any other disease that might involve the pineal organ. It can safely be predicted that their use will enhance our understanding of both pineal tumors and normal pineal function. For example, it does not seem beyond the realm of possibility that the wide range of cell types found among pineal tumors reflects a similar unrecognized heterogeneity in normal pineal organs, and that different types of pineal cells produce different biologically active secretions. If so, each of the subgroups of pineal neoplasms may eventually be found to be associated with its own characteristic pineal hormone pattern. In that event, some future edition of this volume will require an additional chapter.

Richard J. Wurtman, MD
Cambridge, Massachusetts

CHAPTER ONE

Pathology of Tumors of the Pineal Region

Umberto DeGirolami Worcester, Massachusetts

THE CLASSIFICATION OF NEOPLASMS in the region of the pineal gland has evolved along cytogenetic principles. In 1932 del Río-Hortega[1] described two main cell types in the human pineal gland, one with pale nuclei and conspicuous nucleoli, the other with dark nuclei, a homogeneous speckled chromatin, and a stellate cytoplasm. The predominant cells were those with pale nuclei. These were thought to be pineal parenchymal cells. Cells with dark nuclei were interpreted as neuroglial cells, probably of astrocytic origin. Silver carbonate impregnation stained the processes of both cell types and showed clustering of the pineal parenchymal cells in lobules surrounded by astrocytes. With this stain, the specific identifying feature of pineal parenchymal cells was found to be thin cytoplasmic processes ending in club-shaped expansions. Variable numbers of these processes extended towards capillary surfaces.

Krabbe[2, 3] had proposed the inclusive term *pinealoma* for neoplasms arising from the pineal gland and posterior third ventricular region. Horrax and Bailey[4] subdivided tumors of the pineal gland into two groups. The first group, pinealomas, included 11 cases in which the tumor cell type was reminiscent of the adult pineal parenchymal cell. A second group, *teratomas*, included a cystic tumor containing hair, bone, and cartilage. One year later Bailey and Cushing[5] separated the cases of the first group into *pineoblastomas* and *pinealomas*. They defined pineoblastoma as a cellular, rapidly growing tumor of the pineal gland, composed of spongioblasts (ie., primitive glial cells) but without neuroblasts (ie., primitive neurons), stressing its resemblance to the pineal body anlage. The pinealomas were defined as tumors made up of large spherical cells with processes ending in bulbs. The tumor cells in pinealomas were arranged in nests, divided by clusters of small lymphoid cells. Globus and Silbert[6] concluded, from their comparative study of human pineal glands, between the ages of $5\frac{1}{2}$ months gestation to $5\frac{1}{2}$ years, that the various pineal tumors recapitulate human pineal ontogenesis.

1

This view was supported by del Río-Hortega in 1934[7] who thought that pineal tumors adapt a semidifferentiated structure but fail to reach the adult level of differentiation of the pineal parenchyma. Del Río-Hortega defined pineoblastoma as a neoplasm consisting of masses of lymphocyte-like cells forming irregular lobules, which could be outlined by reticulin stains. *Pineocytoma*, a more mature form of the neoplasm, was characterized by its bimorphic pattern of large epitheloid cells disposed in a mosaic among zones of lymphoid-like cells. Baggenstoss and Love[8] added a fifth type of pineal neoplasm to the list, which, by now, included pinealoma, pineocytoma, pineoblastoma, and teratoma, ie., the pineal ependymoma. This neoplasm was characterized by an embryonic row of cuboidal cells, occurring in connection with pineoblastoma.

Russell[9] presented five illustrative cases in support of the thesis that tumors composed of sheets of large spheroid cells (cases 1–4), separated by a connective tissue stroma and infiltrated by lymphocyte-like cells, previously thought to be derived from pineal cells (called both *pinealomas* and *pineocytomas*), were related to teratomas. In the first and second cases the tumor was located in the pineal region; one was associated with a choriocarcinoma and the other with a typical teratoma, both in the pineal. In the third and fourth cases the tumor was restricted to the anterior third ventricle; one was associated with a dermoid cyst of the pineal, the other showed no abnormality in the pineal. In contrast to these four cases, the fifth case seemed to have a fundamentally different histopathology and was characterized by transitions between small and large polygonal cells, with a tendency towards a mosaic arrangement. In this latter case, in distinction to the previous four, silver stains demonstrated club-shaped processes emanating from neoplastic cells, similar to those described by del Río-Hortega[1] as characteristic of normal adult human pineal parenchymal cells. From this case material, Russell[9] concluded that there is a group of intracranial neoplasms with a characteristic histologic picture of large polygonal cells admixed with small lymphocyte-like cells that may be associated with foci of teratoma. Among these, those occurring in the posterior third ventricle (cases 1 and 2) were labeled *atypical teratomas*, reasoning that the neoplasm was the result of differentiation of one predominating cell line rather than three, therefore atypical in its growth. In the same laboratory it had previously been recognized by Professor H. M. Turnbull that this type of tumor of the pineal resembled the spheroidal carcinoma of the testis (seminoma), which had come to be regarded as an atypical teratoma. *Ectopic pinealoma* (cases 3 and 4) was the term used by Russell in this and subsequent publications[10] to refer to cases described by previous reports as pinealomas. In her opinion these tumors were indistinguishable from atypical teratomas, except for their ectopic localization in the anterior third ventricle. Since these four illustrative cases could best be regarded as atypical forms of teratoma and not tumors originating from parenchymal cells of the pineal gland, the older, somewhat indiscriminate designation of these tumors as pinealomas seemed entirely unjustifiable. The neoplasm in the fifth case reported could be demonstrated to show a kinship to the normal adult pineal parenchymal cells and appeared to deserve the designation *true pinealoma*. Friedman[11] reiterated the histologic similarity between seminomas of the testis, dysgerminomas of the ovary, and the pineal atypical teratomas, and introduced *germinoma* as an all-inclusive term for these tumors, be they genital or extragenital in location. Electron microscopic studies of testicular seminomas[12] ovarian dysgerminomas[13–15] ectopic pinealomas and suprasellar germinomas,[16, 17] pineal germinomas, and atypical teratomas[18–22] have confirmed the morphologic similarities between these and identified the lymphocyte-like cells as lymphocytes. It has now become practice in a number of centers[23] to identify all these tumors as germinomas and to qualify the location of the lesion, be it in the testis, ovary, retroperitoneum, mediastinum, suprasellar, intrasellar, or pineal region, where such tumors have been reported to date. Although the designation germinoma is gaining wider acceptance for the pineal neoplasm, the use of the term pinealoma for this tumor is still quite widespread.

Adding to the list of germ-cell tumors of the pineal region that now included typical teratomas and germinomas, several reports have been described recently of neoplasms akin to those recognized in the gonads. As mentioned above, in case 1 of Russell's series[9] there was a *choriocarcinoma* adjacent to a germinoma, and several more recent cases of intracerebral choriocarcinoma are summarized by Rubinstein.[23] Several reports[24–26] have also described another type of germ-cell tumor in the pineal, namely an *embryonal carcinoma*, which in several instances was reminiscent of the endodermal-sinus tumor (yolk-sac carcinoma), as described in the ovary and elsewhere by Teilum.[27] A remarkable case in which a germinoma and an embryonal carcinoma coexisted in the pineal is reported by Jellinger et al.[28]

The tumors of the pineal parenchymal cells were logically included by Russell and Rubinstein[29] under the general heading of pinealomas to reflect the concept described by Russell in 1944 that these are the true pinealomas. A year later, however, it was felt necessary by Rubinstein[23] to delete the term pinealoma altogether and to refer to the true pinealomas as tumors of the pineal parenchyma. Under this heading a more mature form, the pineocytoma, and a more primitive type, the pineoblastoma, were included, reflecting the older terminology mentioned above. Clearly the use of these terms by both Bailey and Cushing,[5] by del Río-Hortega[1, 7] and in a number of other publications in the older literature, does not necessarily identify the neoplasm for the modern reader unless a detailed histopathologic description or a microphotograph accompany the report. A single report on the ultastructure of a pineocytoma[30] compares the structure of the neoplasm to that of the normal adult baboon pineal and to the descriptions of pineals of experimental animals, pointing to several similarities between the tumor and the normal gland. The ultrastructure of the pineocytoma reported by Nielsen and Wilson[30] is quite distinct from that of germinomas reported in several earlier publications. Ultrastructural characteristics of pineoblastomas have not been described to date.

Although the adult human pineal gland does not possess ganglion cells, histogenetic arguments are given by Rubinstein and Okazaki[31] and Rubinstein[32] as to why it would be reasonable to expect the development of neoplasms containing differentiated or undifferentiated elements along neuronal cell lines. One such case, together with the reinterpretation of several earlier cases, is given by Rubinstein and Okazaki.[31] A case of *chemodectoma* in the pineal region is reported by Smith et al.[33]

In view of the extensive recent literature of the neuroendocrine function of the pineal gland in mammalian and nonmammalian species, several interesting points might relate to the diagnostic armamentarium of the future. Several monographs and recent reviews discuss the problem.[34-37] The discovery of melatonin (5-methoxy-N-acetyltryptamine), in 1959, as an indole synthesized only in the pineal, led to a number of experimental studies in nonmammalian species, including the discovery of its skin-lightening action in frogs. It was subsequently observed that in mammalian species the function of melatonin was different and related to inhibition of gonadal development and regulation of estrus. Melatonin is synthesized in the pineal via methylation of N-acetylserotonin by an enzyme found exclusively in the pineal: hydroxyindole-O-methyltransferase (HIOMT). Melatonin, serotonin, and HIOMT have been demonstrated[38] in the subcutaneous metastases of a biopsy proved case of pineal germinoma that had received radiation therapy. Two years later Wurtman and Kammer[39] reported increased synthesis of melatonin in the dural metastases of an autopsy proved case of a germinoma in the anterior third ventricle. There have been no reports to date on the melatonin-forming activity of pineal parenchymal tumors. Since melatonin and melatonin-synthesizing enzymes are held to be derived from the activity of pineal cells, it seems uncertain at the time how best to interpret their presence in the metastases of germ-cell neoplasms. Assays of primary extracranial germinomas would be of interest. Identification of serum or cerebrospinal fluid levels of melatonin-forming activity might form the future basis for diagnosing or discriminating between several diagnostic possibilities in this group of tumors. A pineal-function test has been suggested, based on experimental evidence in rats showing a response to levodopa in the secretions and synthesis of melatonin.

It had been recognized for many years that *gliomas* of varying degrees of malignancy could invade the posterior third ventricle and give rise to a set of signs and symptoms indistinguishable from any other tumors of the pineal gland. A number of reviews and monographs, mainly from neurosurgical clinics, have again emphasized their importance.[40-47] From the diagnostic and therapeutic standpoint, the importance of segregating those gliomas, which by their growth and spread appear to center around the posterior third ventricle and pineal region, has been repeatedly emphasized. Neoplasms arising from the walls of the third ventricle (including thalamic and hypothalamic regions), which manifest early invasion of the cavity of the third ventricle and the rostral mesencephalic region, seem to form one group. The other group consists of neoplasms originating from the glial cells in and around the pineal itself. Although the nomenclature and classification of pineal tumors has undergone considerable renewal over the years, it is still possible to attempt to evaluate the nature of neoplasms described in some of the older literature because of the remarkable clarity of some of these reports. Without exception, the same type of evaluation is exceedingly difficult for the glial-cell neoplasms of the posterior third ventricular region, described in recent reviews. Using the detailed clinical and pathologic descriptions (accompanied by excellent photographs) of the 12 cases of tumors of the pineal body, reported by Horrax and Bailey,[4] it might be possible to reclassify these cases according to contemporary nomenclature as follows: 1 low-grade glioma; 1 pineocytoma; 1 pineoblastoma; 1 teratoma; 6 germinomas; and 2 uncertain types. The case reinterpreted as a low-grade astrocytoma of the pineal was well circumscribed and noninvasive. Five of the 12 cases were noninvasive. In the six cases of astrocytoma and bipolar spongioblastoma, reported by Ringertz et al.[42] in a series of 65 pathologically verified tumors, the bulk of the tumor filled the pineal region and all but one showed invasive features. Of five ependymomas filling the pineal region, two grew infiltratively. The one glioblastoma filled the pineal region and infiltrated both thalami. Of eight autopsy proved gliomas reviewed in a recent series,[48] anaplastic features correlated directly with invasiveness and in one case the neoplasm caused enlargement of the pineal exclusively. This latter case had been discussed by Adams and Richardson[49] as a Cabot case. While at the Armed Forces Institute of Pathology (A.F.I.P) I examined an encapsulated tumor restricted to the pineal having the histopathology of a juvenile pilocytic astrocytoma. Rubinstein[23] accepts a case reported by Zeitlin as an astroblastoma restricted to the pineal. Beyond these cases it is exceedingly difficult to evaluate the pathologic aspects of gliomas of the posterior third ventricle and pineal region. Rand and Lemmen[41] report one *undifferentiated glioma* among 19 pathologically verified cases of posterior third ventricular neoplasm. Cummins et al.[43] described 19 gliomas (13 astrocytomas, 4 ependymomas, and 2 mixed gliomas) in which the bulk of the tumor was almost entirely within the third ventricle and showed limited local invasion, but pathologic details are lacking. Poppen and Marino[45] identify two gliomas among 45 cases. Similarly, among 36 cases of third ventricular tumors reported by Pecker et al.,[44] 12 *benign pedunculated gliomas* are reported, but in this extensive report it is still impossible to grasp the precise nature of these lesions. In spite of the lack of sufficient numbers of well-documented cases of gliomas, confined or arising primarily in the pineal or posterior third ventricular region, it seems entirely reasonable to include these in the classification and to entertain this diagnostic possibility from the clinical, surgical, and radiologic standpoint.

Beyond the three groups of neoplasms of the pineal region mentioned (germ-cell tumors, pineal parenchymal tumors, and gliomas), a variety of neoplasms arising from connective tissue elements, meninges, and blood vessels have been described. Cystic change within the pineal gland, although relatively common in adult pineals examined at autopsy, does occasionally result in obstructive and visual symptoms, necessitating surgical intervention. Well-documented cases are quite rare, although the designation of *cyst* or *arachnoid cyst* is not infrequent in larger series.[46] A case of *hemangiopericytoma* is documented by Olson and Abell.[50] *Melanomas* were recorded in the older literature, but a recent case with proof that the gland is the primary site of the neoplasm is lacking. *Meningiomas* along the meningeal folds of the velum interpositum of sufficient magnitude to present as a posterior third ventricular mass have been recorded by several authors.[51, 52] While there is little doubt that meningiomas can occur in this region and may present a problem of clinical and radiologic differential diagnosis, there is sparse information on the biologic behavior of these lesions.

Cystic change in or about the pineal region may be encountered in association with teratomatous (epidermoid and dermoid) growth within or adjacent to the gland. A recent publication of one such instance refers to nine such instances from the literature.[53] Glial-lined cysts within the pineal are not uncommon at postmortem examination of elderly individuals and have been reported with increased incidence in individuals with systemic cancer.[54] Significant enlargement of these cysts, enough to produce obstruction of the cerebrospinal fluid pathway, was observed by us in the course of reviewing neoplasms of the pineal region, seen at the Massachusetts General Hospital since 1920.[48]

The following classification of pineal and posterior third ventricular tumors is based conceptually on the work of Russell and Rubinstein[29] and Rubinstein,[23] and is intended to reflect cases from the literature cited that have sufficient documentation to merit recognition. A description of the pathologic aspects of the more common types will follow under separate headings. This is based on personally reviewed, published[48] and unpublished, cases and a review of the literature cited.

Classification of Tumors of the Pineal Region

A. Germ Cell Tumors
   1. Germinoma
       a. Posterior third ventricle and pineal
       b. Anterior third ventricle, suprasellar or intrasellar
       c. Combined lesions in anterior and posterior third ventricle, apparently noncontiguous, with or without foci of cystic or solid teratoma.
   2. Teratoma
       a. Evidencing growth along two or three germ lines in varying degrees of differentiation.
       b. Dermoid and epidermoid cysts with or without solid foci of teratoma.
       c. Histologically malignant forms with or without differentiated foci of benign, solid or cystic teratoma—teratocarcinoma, chorioepithelioma, embryonal carcinoma (endodermal-sinus tumor or yolk-sac carcinoma), combinations of these with or without foci of germinoma.

B. Pineal Parenchymal Tumors
   1. Pineocytes
      a. Pineocytoma
      b. Pineoblastoma
      c. Ganglioglioma and chemodectoma
      d. Mixed forms exhibiting transitions between these
   2. Glia
      a. Astrocytoma
      b. Ependymoma
      c. Mixed forms and other less frequent gliomas (glioblastoma, oligo-
         dendroglioma, etc.)
C. Tumors of Supporting or Adjacent Structures
   1. Meningioma
   2. Hemangiopericytoma
D. Non-Neoplastic Conditions of Neurosurgical Importance
   1. "Degenerative" cysts of the pineal lined by fibrillary astrocytes
   2. Arachnoid cysts

Germ Cell Tumors

Germinomas

An excellent review of the pathology of this tumor in 10 new and 104 cases collected from the literature since 1918 is given by Dayan et al.[55] Large series are reported from Japan, where the tumor is more prevalent than elsewhere in the world.[56] Both in the anterior and posterior third ventricular region germinomas are poorly circumscribed, light gray and granular, solid neoplasms, usually about 3 cm in diameter at the time of diagnosis. In posterior third ventricular germinomas, the pineal is often totally destroyed by the tumor (Fig. 1B). Early seeding of the ventricular system and subarachnoid space, together with focal invasion of the walls of the third ventricle and rostral mesencephalon, are almost invariable (Fig. 1A). Occasionally the tumor may spread throughout the ventricular system (Fig. 1D). The incidence of the sites of spread and metastases is given by Dayan et al.[55] Ventricular enlargement secondary to obstruction of the aqueduct or third ventricle is the rule. Hemorrhage into the tumor, necrosis, or cystic degeneration are not found. Our experience is that the tumors are not calcified, though others have reported radiographic evidence of calcification.[43] An extensive review of 58 suprasellar germinomas is given by Camins and Mount.[57] In germinomas in the anterior third ventricle, giving rise to clinical manifestations first referable to this region, the pineal is also found to be the site of neoplasia in only a few cases, when it is systematically studied at autopsy. Rarely these cases have clinical manifestations referable to both the anterior and posterior third ventricle. The question of multicentricity of neoplastic germ cells versus seeding from a posterior or anterior third ventricular germinoma remains sub judice. When the tumor appears to arise in the anterior third ventricle, it tends to fill the floor and invade the walls of the

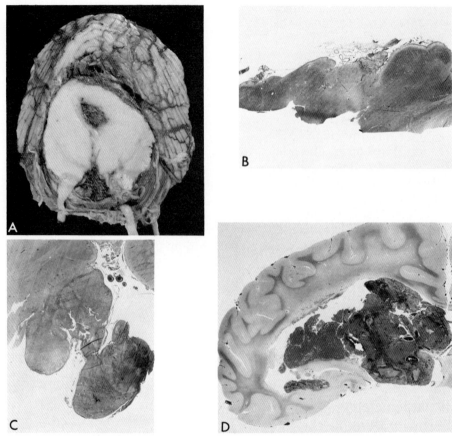

Figure 1A. Pineal germinoma. The tumor invades the quadrigeminal plate and subarachnoid space and totally occludes the aqueduct. **B.** Pineal germinoma. Midsagittal section through diencephalon and rostral brain stem. The tumor destroys the entire pineal gland and invades the quadrigeminal plate (H&E, ×3). **C.** Germinoma in anterior third ventricle (ectopic pinealoma). Midsagittal section through the anterior third ventricle and hypophysis. The tumor extends down to invade the infundibulum and neurohypophysis (H&E, ×3). **D.** Pineal germinoma. Celloidin embedded whole brain coronal section through midparietal region. The tumor fills the lateral ventricles and destroys tissues surrounding the posterior third ventricle (H&E).

ventricle and may extend downward to invade the infundibulum, optic nerves, and pituitary (Fig. 1C). Histologically the tumor is composed of large (15 to 30 μm) cells, with a rounded, centrally placed vesicular nucleus, one or more prominent nucleoli, and abundant clear cytoplasm with distinct cytoplasmic borders (Fig. 2B). These cells tend to form lobules separated by loose connective tissue strands, which are focally infiltrated by clusters of lymphocytes (Fig. 2A). Lymphocytes tend to aggregate around small blood vessels but are not confined to these regions. PAS-positive granules are often present in the cytoplasm of the tumor cells. The Achúcarro-Hortega stain for pineocyte processes is negative.[58] The PTAH stain fails to demonstrate glial

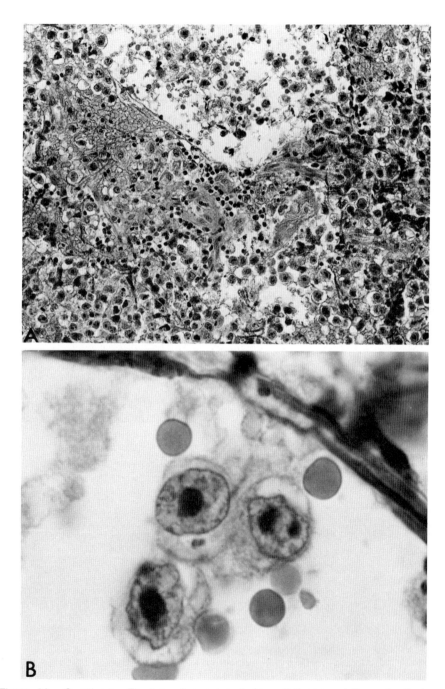

Figure 2A. Germinoma. The tumor is composed of two distinct populations of cells: large, rounded germ cells with prominent nuclei and lymphocytic aggregates (H&E, ×252). **B.** Germinoma. The tumor cell has a rounded vesicular nucleus with prominent nuclear borders and one or more conspicuous nucleoli. The cytoplasmic borders are distinct (H&E, ×1800).

processes in the tumor mass. Mitotic figures are frequent and multinucleated giant cells and frank germinal centers may be seen on occasion. If carefully sought for, foci of teratoma may be found in a number of instances. These most often consist of epithelial-lined portions of cysts or glandular elements. In one case, examined by us with a whole brain section, a focus of epidermoid cysts was found within the tumor in the posterior third ventricle and about a metastatic focus in the frontal horn of the lateral ventricle (Fig. 3D). We would differ with Zülch's[59] interpretation of these tumors, since this and other cases fully support Russell's[9] impression that these tumors are capable of teratomatous growth.

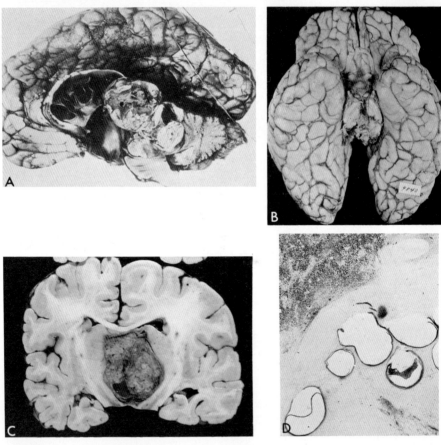

Figure 3A.   Teratoma. Midsagittal brain section. Enormous cystic and solid mass replaces the pineal and displaces midline structures. Note extreme compression of posterior fossa structures. **B.** Teratoma. The tumor has been removed to show destruction of the rostral mesencephalon. **C.** Teratoma. Coronal section through posterior third ventricle. A solid and cystic mass fills the cavity of the third ventricle and compresses adjacent structures. **D.** Teratoma and germinoma. Cysts lined by keratinizing squamous epithelium are found adjacent to a focus of metastatic germinoma in the angle of the lateral ventricle. A germinoma was found in the pineal region (H&E, ×26).

Teratomas

Excellent reviews of the pathology of teratomas of the pineal region are given by Sweet,[60] Walton,[61] Willis,[62] and Tamura et al.[63] Our own experience with well-differentiated teratomas of the pineal region is limited to a very few cases. The tumor may occasionally attain huge proportions (Fig. 3A). It is usually partially encapsulated, noninvasive, lobulated, multicystic, and solid (Fig. 3C). The pineal gland is often totally replaced and the quadrigeminal plate may be destroyed (Fig. 3B). Obstruction of cerebrospinal fluid outflow with symmetrical hydrocephalus is an invariable finding. The presence of radiologic and pathologic evidence of calcification is emphasized in some of the literature but was not present in our cases. The microscopic appearance is that of extracranial teratomas and varies considerably from case to case, oftentimes showing mainly differentiation along ectodermal or mesodermal cell lines. The author is familiar with four unpublished cases of embryonal carcinoma in addition to the ones cited in the literature. In these cases, as in teratocarcinomas in general, the neoplasm is at first locally invasive and then extensively destructive of all tissues around the posterior third ventricle. The histologic features of these exceedingly rare neoplasms are discussed by Bestle,[24] Borit,[25] Jellinger et al.,[28] Rubinstein,[23] and Barlow et al.[26]

Pineal Parenchymal Tumors

Pineocytoma

Of five personally examined cases of pineocytoma, the neoplasm was confined to the posterior third ventricular region in four instances and in one it extended to fill the entire ventricular system as if to form a cast (Fig. 4A). Of the four restricted tumors, the two that came to autopsy showed a pale gray friable mass totally replacing the pineal gland. The outline of the gland could still be distinguished and it appeared as if it were greatly enlarged. The posterior aspect of the tumor was smooth. There was no evidence of extension into the subarachnoid space. The anterior aspect of the tumor projected into the third ventricle, displacing the thalami laterally and the mesencephalon inferiorly (Figs. 5A and C). Even in the case where the neoplasm extended into the ventricle, the outline of an apparently greatly enlarged pineal was still discernible (Fig. 4B). In this instance the tumor in the ventricle had a gray gelatinous appearance. In the case of pineocytoma reported by Dorothy Russell[9] (case 5) the tumor was a partly cystic and partly solid, noninvasive, partially encapsulated mass, which greatly deformed the quadrigeminal plate and projected into the cavity of the third ventricle. The case of pineocytoma reported by Nielsen and Wilson[30] was described at surgery as being light gray, soft, and well circumscribed but not encapsulated. It is difficult to be certain about the precise nature of many of the cases in the older literature. Even in the detailed study of Horrax and Bailey[4] it is not certain whether any of the 12 cases reported are pineocytomas. Dayan et al.[55]

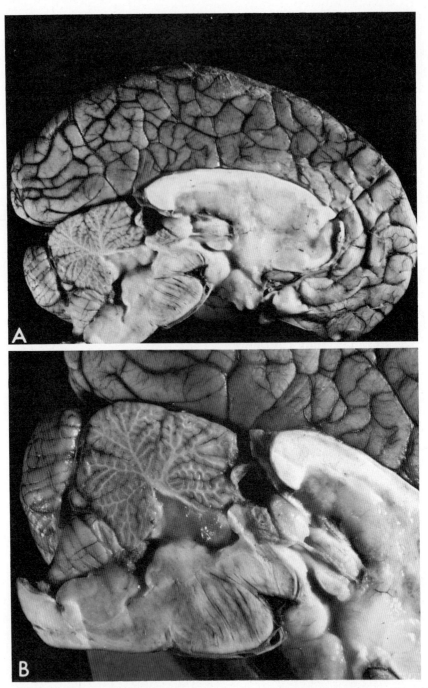

Figure 4A. Pineocytoma (poorly differentiated). Midsagittal section of brain. A gray-white gelatinous tumor fills the entire ventricular system as if to form a cast. **B.** Pineocytoma (poorly differentiated). The pineal gland is uniformly enlarged two to three times its normal size. Note tumor filling the fourth ventricle.

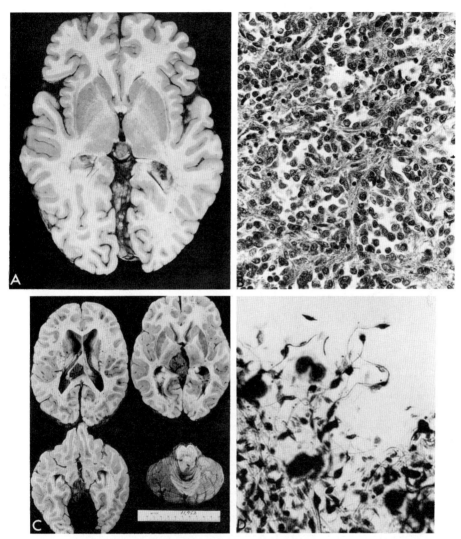

Figure 5A. Pineocytoma (well differentiated). Horizontal section just above pineal recess. The tumor is encapsulated and completely replaces the gland. **B.** Pineocytoma (well differentiated). The resemblance of the tumor to the adult pineal gland is striking. Aggregates of tumor cells varying in size and shape form lobules separated by a thin connective tissue framework. Transition forms between smaller and larger cells are seen (H&E, ×252). **C.** Pineocytoma. Horizontal sections through cerebellum and brain stem. The tumor is largely confined to the posterior third ventricle but is locally invasive. **D.** Pineocytoma (well differentiated). This very high magnification picture shows the tumor cells as blurs. The delicate processes that originate from these end in club-shaped expansions (Modified Achúcarro-Hortega, ×1000).

compare, in chart form, the sites of spread and metastases of 114 atypical teratomas with those of true pineal tumors, but no indication whatever is given as to how these true pineal tumors were selected. Among the seven pineal tumors reported by Globus and Silbert[6] two (cases 5 and 7) can be

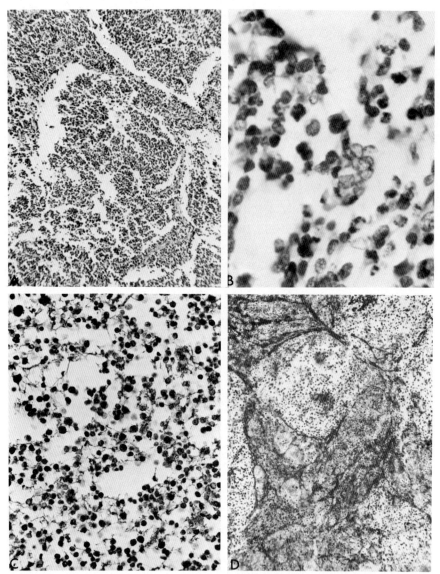

Figure 6A. Pineoblastoma. Densely cellular tumor with little architectural pattern (H&E, ×120). **B.** Pineoblastoma. The tumor cells have hyperchromatic nuclei and scanty cytoplasm. Several mitotic figures are present (H&E, ×750). **C.** Pineoblastoma. Thin and irregular argentophilic cytoplasmic processes are observed (modified Achúcarro-Hortega, ×400). **D.** Pineoblastoma. Reticulin fibers outline lobules giving mosaic pattern (Reticulin, ×160).

interpreted as pineocytoma based on the excellent clinical and pathologic descriptions. One case was well encapsulated and easily separated from the brain substance and the other showed extension of tumor into the lateral ventricle. Based on these cases, it seems reasonable to consider that the majority of pineocytomas are well circumscribed and confined to the posterior

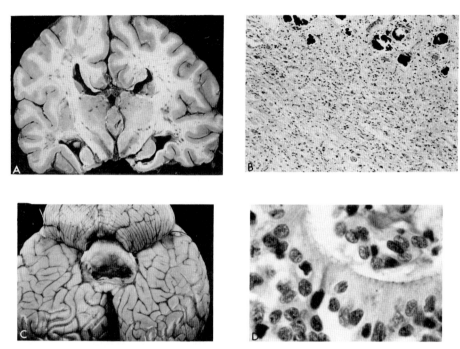

Figure 7A. Astrocytoma (well differentiated). Horizontal section through posterior third ventricle. This very well-circumscribed mass pushes slightly the walls of the third ventricle without invading the brain parenchyma. **B.** Astrocytoma (well differentiated). The tumor is composed of bipolar fibrillary astrocytes. Invasion of normal pineal tissue containing acervuli is noted in the upper right hand corner (H&E, ×200). **C.** Ependymoma. The cerebellum has been lifted and pushed forward to show the tumor in the cavity of the posterior third ventricle. **D.** Ependymoma. Tumor cells with abundant cytoplasm and eccentric nuclei form canals (H&E, ×700).

third ventricle, while some are invasive of the ventricular system and tissue surrounding the posterior third ventricle. This latter group might be expected to show undifferentiated features on histologic examination.

The microscopic picture of pineocytoma is very distinctive. In its mature, differentiated form the neoplasm is almost indistinguishable from the adult pineal gland (Fig. 5B; see also reference 5, cases 5 and 7). The tumor is often moderately cellular and composed of fusiform and rounded cells, with a distinct stellate cytoplasm and round or oval nuclei. The size and shape of the neoplastic cells are not uniform, and varying shapes and sizes may be found within one area. The tumor cells characteristically cluster in *lobules* surrounded by a vascularized connective tissue stroma very much akin to the normal adult human pineal. The nuclei of the neoplastic cells show an even chromatin pattern, often without nucleoli, and vary in staining intensity, depending on the size of the cell. The glial cells seen in the normal pineal are absent from the neoplasm, giving it a more homogeneous and monotonous appearance. The PTAH stain fails to show glial processes. On silver impregnation the tumor cells can be shown to possess the characteristic club-shaped processes originally described by del Río-Hortega in the normal gland.[1] For frozen section preparations, the technique described by Horrax and Bailey[4] is most often used. For paraffin-embedded material, a modification of the original methods of Achúcarro and del Río-Hortega,[58] gives good results. The necessity of running these stains in suspected pineal tumors is emphasized throughout the literature and brought into focus by Russell.[9] The stain is positive only in pineal parenchymal tumors and negative in germ-cell tumors and gliomas. Unfortunately, claims are made in some exhaustive publications in the older literature that club-shaped processes are seen in photographs of neoplasms that look like germinomas to this observer. The cell process that stains with silver impregnation is a slender, sometimes racemose extension from the cell body. It exhibits fusiform swellings along its length and terminates in a club-shaped expansion (Fig. 5D). In a successful impregnation, the delicate processes intertwine as if a thick vine, with the leaves to the sides representing the club-shaped endings. There is a tendency for the processes of normal and neoplastic pineal cells to extend towards capillaries and venules,[1] but they are found elsewhere as well.

Mitotic figures, hemorrhage, necrosis, and calcification are not usually present. In some examples of pineocytoma transition forms between pineoblastoma (see below) and pineocytoma characterize the tumor. In these instances the histology of the lesion is reminiscent of the embryonal pineal gland.[6] The lobular pattern of tumor growth is present, but connective tissue elements are less striking. Individual cells within the lobules are more rounded and have less demonstrable cytoplasm with a more prominent chromatin pattern. Perivascular pseudorosettes and rosettes with central argyrophilic fibers may be seen.

Pineoblastoma

Pineoblastomas are usually frankly invasive, gray-white or reddish-gray, gelatinous tumors that extend into the ventricle and subarachnoid space and are destructive of tissues surrounding the posterior third ventricle. Extension of tumor into the posterior fossa, with involvement of the superior surface of the cerebellum and anterior vermis, is not infrequent and often raises the question of medulloblastoma. In six cases personally reviewed, eight examined by Rubinstein,[32] and four by McGovern,[64] the tumor was frankly invasive, sometimes extending down the neuraxis. Necrosis, hemorrhage, and calcification are not ordinarily observed, while cystic degeneration is observed occasionally. Microscopically the tumor is densely cellular and composed of cells with round or oval nuclei, rich in chromatin, and with scanty irregular cytoplasm (Figs. 6A and B). The presence of rosettes with central argyrophilic fibers is seen in some examples. In these instances the tumor is histologically indistinguishable from medulloblastoma. In some cases a lobular pattern akin to that seen in the fetal pineal is prominent, as the tumor assumes a mosaic pattern with smaller hyperchromatic cells arranged peripherally and larger, better differentiated cells, arranged centrally (Fig.

6D). It is often difficult to demonstrate the characteristic club-shaped processes with silver impregnation of these tumors; however, poorly formed cytoplasmic expansions may be seen if the neoplasm is exhibiting some differentiation towards the center of the lobule (Fig. 6C).

Gliomas

Several examples of well-circumscribed and invasive gliomas of various histologic types are recorded in the literature.[4, 40, 42–45, 48] A well-differentiated astrocytoma may be confined to the pineal (Figs. 7A and B). Ependymomas restricted to the posterior third ventricle have also been observed (Figs. 7C and D). Glioblastomas, ependymomas, low-grade astrocytomas, and oligodendrogliomas have all been observed in this area.

References

1. del Río-Hortega, P., Pineal gland. *Cytology and Cellular Pathology of the Nervous System.* Vol. 2. Edited by W. Penfield. Paul B. Hoeber, New York, 1932, pp. 635–703.
2. Krabbe, K. H., Histologische und Embryologische Untersuchungen über die Zirbeldrüse des Menschen. *Anat Hefte* **54,** 187–319 (1916).
3. Krabbe, K. H., The pineal gland, especially in relation to the problem on its supposed significance in sexual development. *Endocrinology* **7,** 379–414 (1923).
4. Horrax, G. and Bailey, P., Tumors of the pineal body. *Arch. Neurol. Psychiat.* **13,** 423–467 (1925).
5. Bailey, P. and Cushing, H., *A Classification of the Tumors of the Glioma Group on a Histogenetic Basis with a Correlated Study of Prognosis.* J. B. Lippincott, Philadelphia (1926).
6. Globus, J. H. and Silbert, S., Pinealomas. *Arch. Neurol. Psychiat.* **25,** 937–985 (1931).
7. del Río-Hortega, P., *The Microscopic Anatomy of Tumors of the Central and Peripheral Nervous System.* Charles C Thomas, Springfield, Illinois, 1962, pp 18–26.
8. Baggenstoss, A. H. and Love, J. G., Pinealomas. *Arch. Neurol. Psychiat.* **41,** 1187–1206 (1939).
9. Russell, D. S., The pinealoma: its relationship to teratoma. *J. Pathol. Bacteriol.* **56,** 145–150 (1944).
10. Russell, D. S., "Ectopic pinealoma": its kinship to atypical teratoma of the pineal gland. Report of a case. *J. Pathol. Bacteriol.* **68,** 125–129 (1954).
11. Friedman, N. B., Germinoma of the pineal. Its identity with germinoma ("seminoma") of the testis. *Cancer Res.* **7,** 363–368 (1947).
12. Pierce, G. B., Ultrastructure of human testicular tumors. *Cancer* **19,** 1963–1983 (1966).
13. Lynn, J. A., Varon, H. H., Kingsley, W. B. and Martin, J. H., Ultrastructural and biochemical studies of estrogen secretory capacity of a "non-functional" ovarian neoplasm (dysgerminoma). *Am. J. Pathol.* **51,** 639–661 (1967).
14. Kay, S., Silverberg, S. G. and Schatzki, P. F., Ultrastructure of an ovarian dysgerminoma. *Am. J. Clin. Pathol.* **58,** 456–468 (1972).
15. Hou-Jensen, K. and Kempson, R. L., The ultrastructure of gonadoblastoma and dysgerminoma. *Hum. Pathol.* **5,** 79–91 (1974).
16. Misugi, K., Liss, L. and Bradel, E. J., Electron microscopic study of an ectopic pinealoma. *Acta Neuropathol.* **9,** 346–356 (1967).
17. Hirano, A., Llena, J. F. and Chung, H. D., Some new observations in an intracranial germinoma. *Acta Neuropathol.* **32,** 103–113 (1975).
18. Ramsey, H. J., Ultrastructure of a pineal tumor. *Cancer* **18,** 1014–1025 (1965).
19. Cravioto, H. and Dart, D., The ultrastructure of "pinealoma". *J. Neuropathol. Exp. Neurol.* **32,** 552–565 (1973).

20. Tabuchi, K., Yamada, O. and Nishimoto, A., The ultrastructure of pinealomas. *Acta Neuropathol.* **24,** 117–127 (1973).
21. Tani, E., Ikeda, K., Kudo, S., Yamagata, S., Nishiura, M. and Higashi, N., Specialized intercellular junctions in human intracranial germinomas. *Acta Neuropathol.* **27,** 139–151 (1974).
22. Markesbery, W. R., Brooks, W. H., Milsow, L. and Mortara, R. H., Ultrastructural study of the pineal germinoma in vivo and in vitro. *Cancer* **37,** 327–337 (1976).
23. Rubinstein, L. J., *Tumors of the Central Nervous System,* Atlas of Tumor Pathology, Second Series, Fasc 6. Armed Forces Institute of Pathology, Washington, DC, 1972, pp. 269–284.
24. Bestle, J., Extragonadal endodermal sinus tumours originating in the region of the pineal gland. *Acta Pathol. Microbiol. Scand.* **74,** 214–222 (1968).
25. Borit, A. Embryonal carcinoma of the pineal region. *J. Pathol.* **97,** 165–168 (1969).
26. Barlow, C. F., Richardson, E. P. and Robboy, S. J., Case 41-1974. Endodermal-sinus tumor originating in region of pineal gland, involving hypothalamus, with metastases to spinal cord. *N. Engl. J. Med.* **291,** 837–843 (1974).
27. Teilum, G., *Special Tumors of Ovary and Testis, and Related Extragonadal Lesions.* J. B. Lippincott, Philadelphia (1971).
28. Jellinger, K., Minauf, M., Kraus, H. and Sunder-Plassmann, M., Embryonales Carcinom der Epiphysenregion. *Acta Neuropathol.* **15,** 176–182 (1970).
29. Russell, D. S. and Rubinstein, L. J., *Pathology of Tumors of the Nervous System.* Third edition. Edward Arnold, London, 1971, pp 308–320.
30. Nielsen, S. L. and Wilson, C. B., Ultrastructure of a "pineocytoma". *J. Neuropathol. Exp. Neurol.* **34,** 148–158 (1975).
31. Rubinstein, L. J. and Okazaki, H., Gangliogliomatous differentiation in a pineocytoma. *J. Pathol.* **102,** 27–32 (1970).
32. Rubinstein, L. J., Cytogenesis and differentiation of primitive central neuroepithelial tumors. *J. Neuropathol. Exp. Neurol.* **31,** 7–26 (1972).
33. Smith, W. T., Hughes, B. and Ermocilla, R., Chemodectoma of the pineal region, with observations on the pineal body and chemoreceptor tissue. *J. Pathol. Bacteriol.* **92,** 69–76 (1966).
34. Wurtman, R. J., Axelrod, J. and Kelly, D. E., *The Pineal.* Academic Press, New York (1968).
35. *The Pineal Gland.* Edited by G.E.W. (Wolstenholme, J.) Knight, Churchill-Livingstone, Edinburgh, 1971.
36. Editorial: The pineal. Lancet, November 23, 1974, pp 1235–1237.
37. Axelrod, J., The pineal gland: a neurochemical transducer. *Science* **184,** 1341–1348 (1974).
38. Wurtman, R. J., Axelrod, J. and Toch. R., Demonstration of hydroxyindole-*O*-methyl transferase, melatonin and serotonin in a metastatic parenchymatous pinealoma. *Nature* **204,** 1323–1324 (1964).
39. Wurtman, R. J. and Kammer, H., Melatonin synthesis by an ectopic pinealoma. *N. Engl. J. Med.* **274,** 1233–1237 (1966).
40. Dandy, W. E., *Benign Tumors of the Third Ventricle.* Charles C Thomas, Springfield, Illinois, 1933.
41. Rand, R. W. and Lemmen, L. J., Tumors of the posterior portion of the third ventricle. *J. Neurosurg.* **10,** 1–18 (1953).
42. Ringertz, N., Nordenstam, H. and Flyger, G., Tumors of the pineal region. *J. Neuropathol. Exp. Neurol.* **13,** 540–561 (1954).
43. Cummins, F. M., Taveras, J. M. and Schlesinger, E. B., Treatment of gliomas of the third ventricle and pinealomas; with special reference to the value of radiotherapy. *Neurology* **10,** 1031–1036 (1960).
44. Pecker, J., Ferrand, B. and Javalet, A., Tumeurs du triosième ventricule. *Neurochirurgie* **12,** 1–136 (1969).

45. Poppen, J. L. and Marino, R., Pinealomas and tumors of the posterior portion of the third ventricle. *J. Neurosurg.* **28,** 357–364 (1968).
46. Stein, B. M., The infratentorial supracerebellar approach to pineal lesions. *J. Neurosurg.* **35,** 197–202 (1971).
47. Stein, R. M., Fraser, R. A. R. and Tenner, M. S., Tumours of the third ventricle in children. *J. Neurol. Neurosurg. Psychiat.* **35,** 776–788 (1972).
48. DeGirolami, U. and Schmidek, H., Clinicopathological study of 53 tumors of the pineal region. *J. Neurosurg.* **39,** 455–462 (1973).
49. Adams, R. D. and Richardson, E. P. Case 38521. Pinealoma, astrocytomatous form. *N. Engl. J. Med.* **247,** 1036–1040 (1952).
50. Olson, J. R. and Abell, M. R., Haemangiopericytoma of the pineal body. *J. Neurol. Neurosurg. Psychiat.* **32,** 445–449 (1969).
51. Araki, C., Meningioma in the pineal region; a report of two cases, removed by operation. *Arch. Jap. Chir.* **14,** 1181–1192 (1937).
52. Sachs, E., Avman, N. and Fisher, R., Meningiomas of the pineal region and posterior part of the 3rd ventricle. *J. Neurosurg.* **19,** 325–331 (1962).
53. Sambasivan, M. and Nayar, A., Epidermoid cyst of the pineal region. *J. Neurol. Neurosurg. Psychiat.* **37,** 1333–1335 (1974).
54. Hajdu, S. I., Porro, R. S., Lieberman, P. H. and Foote, F. W., Degeneration of the pineal gland of patients with cancer. *Cancer* **29,** 706–709 (1972).
55. Dayan, A. D., Marshall, A. H. E., Miller, A. A., Pick, F. J. and Rankin, N. E., Atypical teratomas of the pineal and hypothalamus. *J. Pathol. Bacteriol.* **92,** 1–28 (1966).
56. Susuzki, J. and Iwabuchi, T., Surgical removal of pineal tumors (pinealomas and teratomas). Experience in a series of 19 cases. *J. Neurosurg.* **23,** 565–571 (1965).
57. Camins, M. B., and Mount, L. A., Primary suprasellar atypical teratoma. *Brain* **97,** 447–456 (1974).
58. De Girolami, U. and Zvaigzne, O., Modification of the Achúcarro-Hortega pineal stain for paraffin-embedded formalin-fixed tissue. *Stain Technol.* **48,** 48–50 (1973).
59. Zülch, K. J., *Brain Tumors. Their Biology and Pathology.* Second edition. Springer, New York, 1965, p 189.
60. Sweet, W. H., A review of dermoid, teratoid and teratomatous intracranial tumours. *Dis. Nerv. Syst.* **1,** 228–238 (1940).
61. Walton, K., Teratomas of the pineal region and their relationship to pinealomas. *J. Pathol. Bacteriol.* **61,** 11–21 (1949).
62. Willis, R. A., *Teratomas,* Atlas of Tumor Pathology, Sect. 3, Fasc 9. Armed Forces Institute of Pathology, Washington, DC. (1951).
63. Tamura, H., Kury, G. and Suzuki, K., Intracranial teratomas in fetal life and infancy. *Obstet. Gynecol.* **27,** 134–141 (1966).
64. McGovern, J. V., Tumors of the epiphysis cerebri. *J. Pathol. Bacteriol.* **61,** 1–9 (1949).

CHAPTER TWO

The Neuro-Ophthalmic and Neurologic Manifestations of Pinealomas

Shirley H. Wray Boston, Massachusetts

TUMORS OF THE PINEAL region and ectopic pinealomas, although relatively rare, have always intrigued neurologists, neurosurgeons, and ophthalmologists because of the ocular signs they produce and the complexity of their management.

This chapter reviews the neuro-ophthalmic and neurologic manifestations of pinealomas. The neuroanatomy and pathophysiology of the visual and oculomotor systems affected by these tumors are discussed. Emphasis is also placed on methods of examination and clinical findings that indicate beginning dysfunction. Pinealoma cases taken from the author's files and the Massachusetts General Hospital series are reviewed in detail.

Pineal Region Tumors

Paralysis of Vertical Gaze

Upward gaze palsy is the most common neuro-ophthalmic manifestation of a tumor in the region of the pineal gland (Table 1, Fig. 8). The paresis initially appears to selectively affect upward saccades, but if pursuit function is tested correctly, it is always affected and vertical opticokinetic nystagmus (OKN) responses are also abnormal. The presence of vertical eye movement with neck flexion, simultaneous bilateral caloric stimulation with hot or cold water, and the Bell's phenomenon (Fig. 9) are evidence that the palsy is supranuclear in origin. But, it is noteworthy that not all patients with

Associate Professor of Neurology, Harvard Medical School,
Boston, Massachusetts

Table 1.   Ocular Symptoms and Signs in 22 Cases of Pinealoma

		No. of patients
Symptoms	Diplopia	7
	"Blurred vision"	4
	Reading difficulty	1
Signs	Upward gaze palsy	12
	Pupils: Areflexic to light, near response retained	13
	Accommodative control disorder	3
	Convergent-retraction nystagmus	10
	Convergence paretic	3
	Downward gaze palsy	0
	Collier's sign	0
	Skew deviation	5
	Third nerve palsy	0
	Fourth nerve palsy (bilateral)	1
	Sixth nerve palsy	3
	Fundi: Normal	8
	Papilledema	10
	Optic atrophy	4
	Vision: Reduced acuity	8
	Visual fields: Normal	15
	Constricted	3
	Bitemporal	4

vertical gaze palsy from pinealoma have normal vestibulo-ocular responses or Bell's reflex.[1, 2]

Sustained gaze-evoked upbeat nystagmus rarely precedes the limitation of voluntary upward movement. Pontine lesions involving the tegmentum bilaterally may produce an acute upward gaze palsy that characteristically improves, with only gaze-evoked nystagmus remaining. In these cases a coexisting horizontal gaze palsy persists. Vertical gaze-evoked upbeat nystagmus is also a common sign with bilateral internuclear ophthalmoplegia.

The innervational disturbances responsible for the absence of upward saccades and smooth pursuit in dorsal lesions of the rostral midbrain have been studied.[3-7] Ocular electromyographic (EMG) studies of attempted upward pursuit demonstrate impaired facilitation of the agonist elevator muscles and failure of the antagonist depressor muscles to inhibit. The eyes are thus prevented from elevating by an inhibitory failure. This mechanism is considered analogous to the pathophysiology of horizontal gaze palsies.[7] During attempted upward saccades, a phasic anomaly accompanies contraction of all extraocular muscles, resulting in retraction nystagmus.[4]*

---

* A monocular supranuclear upward gaze palsy with retention of the Bell's reflex can occur in pretectal or periaqueductal disease.[14-17] The eyes are straight in the primary position and only move disconjunctively as the patient looks upward. Monocular supranuclear upward gaze palsy is due to a discrete lesion, usually vascular, in the pretectal region close to the contralateral oculomotor nucleus involving both crossed and uncrossed central neural connections to the subnuclei of the superior rectus and inferior oblique muscles.[16] A case report of a single brain-stem metastasis confirmed the site and side of the rostral midbrain lesion.[17]

Caution should be exercised in predicting a poor prognosis for recovery of upward gaze in pineal region tumors. Full-gaze movements may be restored simply by relieving pressure on the pretectum following a shunt operation for

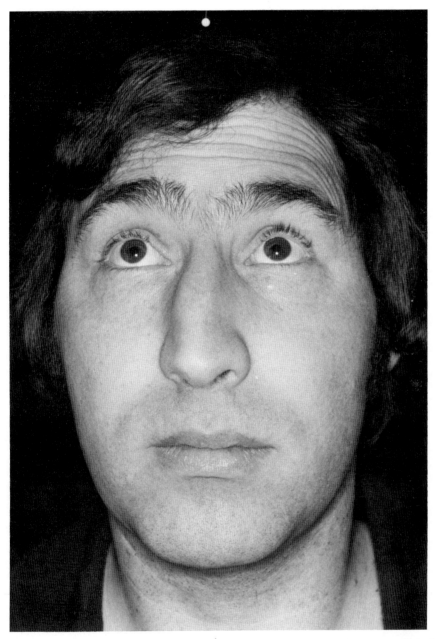

Figure 8 Paralysis of upward gaze in 27-year-old man with a pineal region tumor. Note the elevation of the eyebrows and innervation of the frontalis with wrinkling of the forehead (Case 7).

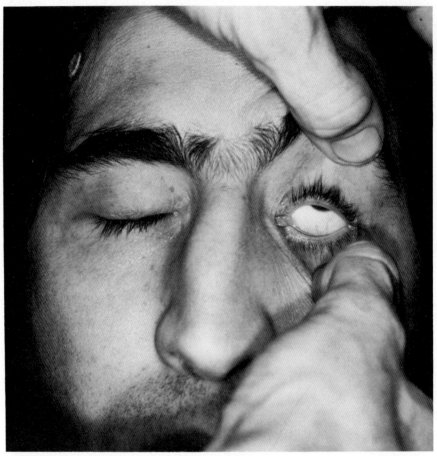

Figure 9   Intact Bell's reflex in the patient shown in Figure 8 with a supranuclear upward gaze plasy. The eyes during forced eyelid closure show upward tonic deviation.

hydrocephalus.[8] (See also references 9–13 for information on the pathophysiology of vertical gaze paresis as a *false* localizing sign in acute obstructive hydrocephalus.)

Isolated downward gaze palsy in pineal region tumors is rare. When this sign does occur, it affects both saccadic and pursuit movements and is associated with upward gaze and convergence paresis. It implies involvement of the anterior mesencephalon.

A systematic ocular motility examination is necessary to facilitate the early detection of impaired upward gaze. The functional importance to the clinician of the tripartite division of eye movements into saccades, smooth pursuit, and vestibular movements is reemphasized.

Observe first the position of the head and eyes at rest. Displacement of the eyes below the horizontal meridian occurs with an acute palsy of upward gaze. This sign, frequently subtle, is of particular value in the examinaton of the comatose or obtunded patient. The alert standing patient with a complete upward gaze palsy may adopt a compensatory *head-back* posture.

To test voluntary vertical saccades (command or schematic saccades), ask the patient to look up and down. Command saccades can be made in the dark or in light. The movement is internally programmed without a target or parafoveal image. The amplitude of the voluntary upward movement should be at least 30°. The maximum range of upward gaze diminishes with age, so that by the seventh decade it may be restricted to 15°.[18] Paralytic and slow, voluntary, upward saccades are best observed with the patient sitting erect, facing the examiner. Absence of *voluntary* saccades can only be confirmed when the patient is *trying* to make *schematic* upward eye movements.

To test refixation vertical saccades, ask the patient to change fixation and look up to a second point in space. This saccade requires attention, or shift of attention, and takes about 200 msec for programming and execution. It is not strictly *voluntary*, or it need not be. A single upward refixation saccade or *flick* of the eyes from down gaze to the midposition is a trick that, with only rare exception, will routinely expose the convergent jerks of convergent-retraction nystagmus. It is the best bedside method in Hoyt's experience.[19]

Reflex saccades are evoked by a lower level (nonvisual) sensory input, i.e., from vestibular end organs, neck proprioceptors, or spontaneously, as in sleep, myoclonic central discharge, epilepsy, and vestibular nystagmus, and by fast-moving opticokinetic nystagmus (OKN) stimuli. Optocokinetic nystagmus is an extremely complex reflex response triggered by a particular visual input. Vertical OKN testing is an easy way to show that *reflex* saccades are present or absent. Rotation down of a moving stripe (or object) in front of the eyes produces slow movement of the eyes in the same direction, which, for clinical expedience, is considered a slow-phase pursuit movement. A rapid compensatory movement in the opposite direction, the fast phase, is a corrective saccade that rapidly refixates the eye to the next target. Clinically, vertical OKN is evoked by the use of an OKN tape or drum, which utilizes contrasting alternating squares, stripes, or patterns (Fig. 10). The OKN response depends on visual acuity sufficient to see the stimuli, and, if necessary, the patient should wear his glasses to ensure good fixation. Loss of reflex saccades is confirmed by noting the absence of saccades in the rapid eye movement phase of sleep. By bilateral caloric testing the absence of vestibular evoked saccades, ie., fast phase of vestibular nystagmus, can be confirmed.

To test pursuit eye movements instruct the patient to fix continuously on a target moved slowly in vertical and horizontal directions. The target should be held at least 3 ft in front of the patient to minimize convergence. The extent of full down gaze is inspected with the lids held elevated. In the normal alert patient tracking movements are executed smoothly, but saccadic pursuit (cogwheel eye movements) can be a normal form or mode of pursuit used when the patient is tired and when the object moves irregularly or too rapidly for the system. Some saccadic corrections occur in all attempts to make continuous smooth pursuit. Also, pursuit movements can become saccadic when the patient is unable to generate continuous smooth movement while looking at a sinusoidally moving target. This low-gain pursuit output is, in a sense, a partial palsy of smooth pursuit control. This pursuit disorder occurs when alertness, attention, calibration of retinal velocity or efference signal is impaired. Saccadic pursuit is the earliest eye sign in patients taking anticonvulsants or sedatives.

Patients with absent upward saccadic and pursuit movements show, on attempted upward gaze, elevation of the eyebrows and innervation of the frontalis with wrinkling of the forehead (Fig. 8), a useful point of distinction, since in hysterical *paralysis* of upward gaze the brows usually remain stationary. Also observe whether the eyes are equally limited. Small vertical differences in eye position are the rule, even though diplopia is frequently absent. If the observations are confusing, the motility of each eye is examined alone. (See comment on skew deviation.)

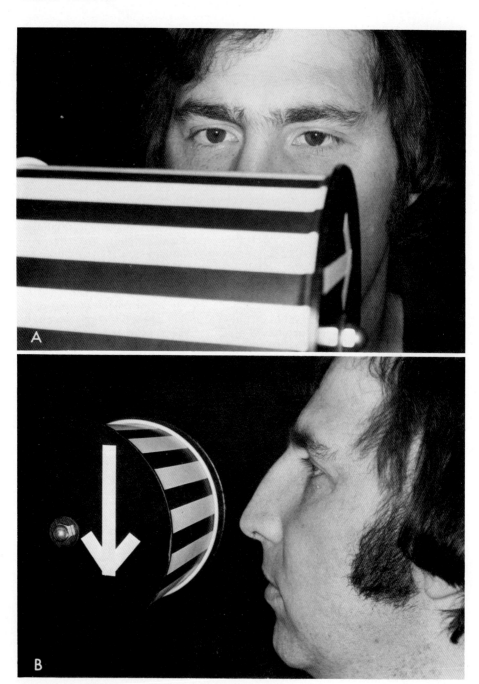

Figure 10 **A.** Vertical optokinetic nystagmus, one method to show that "reflex" saccades are present or absent. The striped drum is rotated with the lines going down (see also Fig. 16). **B.** The technique is used to elicit convergent-retraction nystagmus in patients with the sylvian aqueduct syndrome.

The examination of the oculocephalic reflex (doll's head movements or the Roth-Bielschowsky deviation) is important when a complete vertical palsy is present.[8] The technique is simple. The head is rapidly passively flexed and extended, with the eyes held open (obtunded patient), or fixed (alert patient) on the examiner's nose. Depression of the chin reflexely produces conjugate upward deviation, elevation of the chin, and depression of the eyes. Intact oculocephalic reflexes indicate the integrity of the brainstem tegmentum and the final common pathways for eye movement.

Bilateral caloric stimulation by simultaneous irrigation of the ears with warm or cold water is required to produce vertical ocular deviation. For this reason, and for certain technical considerations, the procedure is rarely performed at the bedside in an alert patient. If the test is required, the most reliable result will be obtained with the patient sitting erect. Bilateral simultaneous irrigation of the external auditory canals with 250 ml of cold water (30°C or ice water for maximal stimulation) for 60 seconds produces conjugate tonic downward deviation of the eyes with the fast phase of the nystagmus upwards. Bilateral simultaneous irrigation with 250 ml of warm water (44°C) for 60 seconds induces tonic upward deviation with the rapid phase of the evoked nystagmus downward. Vertical movements result because sensory evoked signals from the lateral semicircular canals cancel. Changing the temperature of the water reverses the direction of flow of endolymph within the canals and changes the pressure gradient across the cupula. Simultaneous bilateral ear stimulation, with the eyes in the primary position, also cancels out the rotary component that would be seen if only one ear is irrigated. Bilateral simultaneous cold-water caloric stimulation, producing upbeat nystagmus, is one way to elicit *convergent-retraction* jerks of the eyes of a patient with a pineal region tumor.

Bell's phenomenon, the upward (or upward and outward) tonic deviation of the eyes during forced lid closure, may also be observed.[8] Ask the patient to squeeze his eyes shut for several seconds and then note the corrective downward movement of the eyes as the lids open. Intact Bell's phenomenon in a patient with a voluntary upward gaze paresis is evidence of dissociation in upgaze innervation and a supranuclear type of palsy* (Fig. 9). Data available from experimental lesions in animals suggest that an intact frontomesencephalic gaze mechanism is a prerequisite for this reflex ocular deviation.

Paralysis of Pupils and Accommodation

With paralysis of upward gaze, with rare exception pupillary reflexes are abnormal (Table 1). Gowers[20] was the first to report pupillary areflexia and upgaze palsy from a pathologically confirmed pinealoma. Interestingly, in Parinaud's[21] report 2 years later, the pupils were small and recorded as nonreactive to convergence, while light reactions were retained. In our experience, and in the reports of others,[2, 22–24] light-near dissociation of pupillary light reflexes occurs frequently. The pupils are moderately dilated and fixed, or poorly reactive to direct light stimulation while pupillary constriction with the near reflex is retained (Figs. 11A and B). This type of pupil abnormality has been called Argyll-Robertson pupils, but it differs from classic Argyll-Robertson pupils by virtue of lack of miosis and the normal response to atropine. The afferent fibers of the pupillary light reflex pass from the optic tract to the pretectum, where they decussate, in part, through the

---

* See note of caution as to the reliability of this sign, vide supra.

posterior commissure before reaching reticular cells surrounding the Edinger-Westphal nucleus. Light reflex abnormality is frequently present in patients with pineal area tumors. Control signals for accommodation come from the striate and peristriate cortex, traverse the posterior capsule, and reach the Edinger-Westphal nucleus from below[25] (Fig. 12). Pineal region tumors may result in a state of spastic-paretic accommodation. When gaze is shifted from distance to near, accommodation is paretic; on attempted upward gaze accommodative spasms occur, such that distant vision is blurred due to momentary myopia. Importantly, Walsh and Hoyt[26] have observed disorder of accommodative control and pupillary dilation with loss of response to light as the initial signs of pineal tumor weeks before they could record a limited upward gaze. Electronic infrared pupillographic studies have now shown that pineal region tumors impair both light and near responses and that true *light-near dissociation* is rare.[27]

Impaired sympathetic pupillary control is equally rare. Consequently anisocoria has usually been ascribed to asymmetric parasympathetic motor neuron involvement. But, recent observations suggest some patients may have partial central sympathetic impairment and that changes in pupil size are related to the relative imbalance between these two opposing autonomic systems.[28]

While paralysis of upward gaze with retention of normal pupillary reflexes does occur with some pineal region tumors, including invasive thalamic gliomas, mention should also be made of a pupillary syndrome of the anterior midbrain, alternating contraction anisocoria.[28] This is characterized by greater pupillary constriction in the directly stimulated eye than in the consensually reacting pupil which may be a sign of minimal pretectal impairment. Also rarely, Parinaud's syndrome may be associated with corectopia or displaced pupil, which may be permanent or transient.[29] Recently a case of midbrain corectopia has been described in a patient with bilateral rostral midbrain infarction.[30] The pupils were noted to dilate spontaneously, independently, and eccentrically (Fig. 13). Sporadic cycles of dilation and constriction, each lasting 5 to 15 minutes, occurred during the last 3 days of the patient's life. The aperture expanded irregularly to an oval shape. The pupils independently shifted off-center, upward and outward in the right eye and downward and outward in the left eye. The pupils reconstricted, became round, and returned to the center. Autopsy in this case disclosed isolated but intact Edinger-Westphal nuclei. An explanation of midbrain corectopia by the authors centered on the segmental innervation of the pupil by the Edinger-Westphal nucleus. In the presence of a paralyzed dilator muscle, select, central inhibition of sphincter tone resulted in oval and eccentric pupils.

Measurements of pupil size are made in room light, in dim light, and with the patient looking at near. To determine anisocoria pupil diameters are measured with the pupils illuminated obliquely from below. While size is assessed, inequalities in pupil shape and position are noted. Light reactivity in each eye is tested, using a bright light source and observing the rapidity and

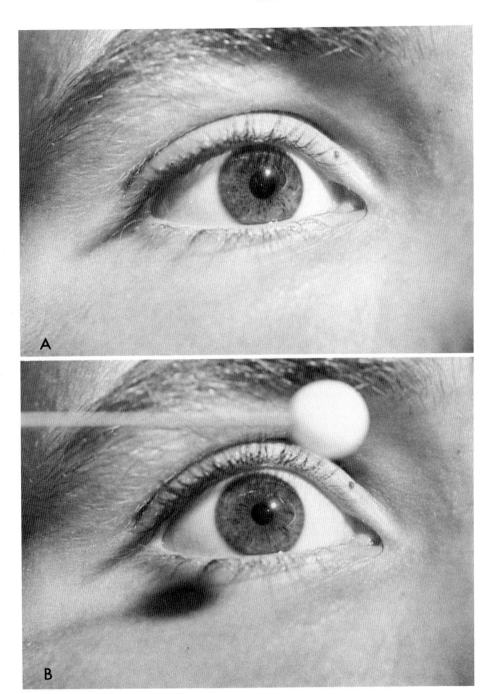

Figure 11   A. Pupillary areflexia to light. **B.** Pupillary constriction with the near reflex. The patient, a 21-year-old man with an epidermoid cyst of the pineal region (Case 13) was asked to focus on a near target (white pinhead) placed directly in front of the eye.

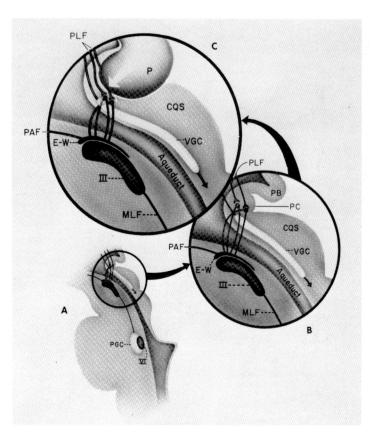

Figure 12   Hypothetical diagram of the tectal area of a patient with a pineal region tumor. The pupillary fibers for accommodation appear to come from below and are initially spared with a compressive lesion from above. **A.** Normal lateral brain stem view. **B.** Normal tectal anatomy. **C.** Pineal region tumor distorting tectal anatomy. CQS = corpus quadrigeminus superior; E-W = Edinger-Westphal nucleus; MLF = medial longitudinal fasciculus; P = pineal region tumor; PAF = afferent pupillary accommodative fibers; PB = pineal body; PC = posterior commissure; PGC = pontine gaze center; PLF = afferent pupillary light fibers; VGC = vertical gaze "center." (Reproduced by permission from Gay, A. T., Newman, N. M., Keltner, J. L., et al.: *Eye Movement Disorders.* C. W. Mosby, St. Louis, 1974).

degree of constriction as well as the size sustained. The direct-light reaction should equal the consensual in every parameter. The pretectal nuclear complex in the rostrodorsal midbrain cannot differentiate which retina is being illuminated, and the efferent impulse sent to both pupillary sphincters is equal.

To test the near response the patient is asked to fix on a near target and the degree of miosis is noted. When paresis of convergence is present, a near response of the pupil can be demonstrated by asking the patient to focus on a near target placed directly in front of the eye (Fig. 11B). Pupil size must also be noted if *spasms* of convergence or convergent-retraction nystagmus occurs.

The accommodative power of the eye is measured in terms of near point (the shortest distance from the naked eye at which an accommodative target can no longer be focused and appears blurred), or the power of minus lenses the eye can overcome. With the latter technique the best corrected distance acuity may be used.

Paralysis of Convergence

Paralysis of convergence is the third sign completing the triad of Parinaud's syndrome.[21, 31] The syndrome of convergence palsy is characterized by a failure of convergence with crossed diplopia when the eyes view a near target but with absence of paresis of the medial recti on lateral gaze. Although the anatomic substrates for convergence, vertical gaze, and pupillary reactions lie in the same vicinity in the midbrain, convergence is often retained when only upward gaze is involved (Table 1). Convergence is usually absent when downward gaze palsy is added.

Convergent jerks of the eyes may occur in patients with upgaze palsy from pineal region tumors. The convergent movements are rapid and are evoked by maximum effort to look upward. This rare type of spasm may be associated with miosis, but this is not invariable.[32, 33] In the cases seen by the author miosis was not present. Paroxysmal convergent movements and defective pupillary light reaction also occur.[34]

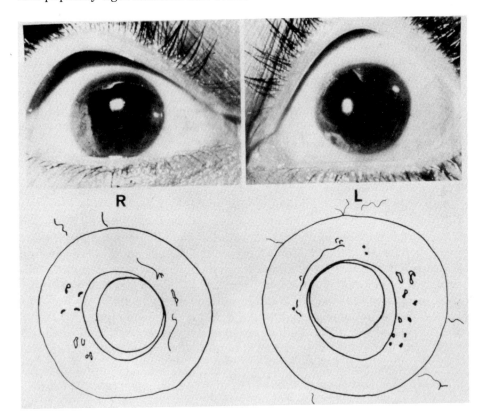

Figure 13   Midbrain corectopia. **Top,** right pupil (R) is in miotic phase and left pupil (L) is in corectopic phase. **Bottom,** limits of both phases of each pupil are depicted. Paired irregular markings on the iris drawings indicate central to peripheral shift of iris crypts during change from miotic to corectopic postions of pupils. (Reproduced by permission from Selhorst, J. B., Hoyt, W. F., Feinsod, M., et al.: Midbrain corectopia. *Arch. Neurol.* **33,** 193–195 (1976)).

The convergence spasm with pineal tumors should not be confused with spasm of the near reflex, which occurs as a functional abnormality.[35–37*]

> To recognize a convergence defect the patient is asked to fix on an object (eg., the patient's own wristwatch) rapidly brought in towards the nose. Alertness and good fixation effort are important. Pupillary constriction indicates that *near* effort is being made (Fig. 14). The normal near point of convergence in the young adult is 70 mm or less; that is, the point where one or both of the converging eyes breaks fixation and turns out. If complete paralysis of convergence is present, the eyes remain immovable.

Convergent-Retraction Nystagmus and Myoclonic Ocular Phenomena

Classic descriptions of the sylvian aqueduct syndrome report an associated range of phenomena, including pure retraction nystagmus (nystagmus retractorius), pure convergent nystagmus, and the two combined.[38–44] Barany[45] reported a case with unilateral retraction nystagmus associated with convergent nystagmus of the contralateral eye. Both phenomena have been reported to occur intermittently in the same eye with lesions in the rostral midbrain.[46]

Convergent-retraction nystagmus is perhaps the most distinctive pretectal phenomenon produced by pineal region tumors. Convergent-retraction nystagmus may be present before upward gaze becomes grossly limited. With every attempt to make an upward saccade, the eyes first jerk inward (Fig. 15) several times, then diverge again. When the phenomenon is pronounced, any saccadic attempt, horizontal or vertical, causes a convergent jerk of the eyes followed by a slower divergent drift back to the parallel position. Attempts to make vertical saccades that produce instead bursts of low-amplitude, rapid eye movement have been called *lightning movements* by Atkin and Bender.[47] Patients with such signs complain of slowness in focusing and difficulty in reading. When convergent eye movements distort horizontal saccades, the resulting limited abduction mimics partial abducens nerve palsy, so called *pseudoabducens palsy* of upper midbrain lesions.[1] Oculocephalic or caloric stimulation usually produces full abduction and thereby resolves the question of paresis. Convergent-retraction nystagmus also occurs on attempted convergence and refocusing on a nearby object, on attempted downward saccades,[2] and spontaneously as a paroxysmal burst of motor activity.[44] The presence or absence of retraction is best detected by viewing the patient's eye from the side (Figs. 10 and 16). Retraction nystagmus is not as well sustained as the usual types of nystagmus and is related to effort on attempted upward gaze.

> The best and simplest bedside test to elicit convergent-retraction nystagmus is to ask the patient to make an upward saccade, or *flick* the eyes, to the midposition[19] (viz supra). The movement invariably evokes convergent jerks. The OKN drum, with downgoing targets, is also a very effective way to elicit

---

* If divergence paralysis occurs in pineal region tumors, the condition is associated with increased intracranial pressure. The patients are orthophoric at near but manifest a concomitant esotropia at distance.

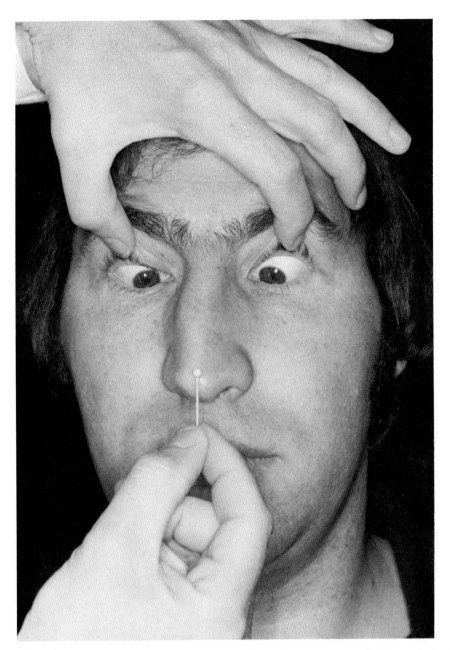

Figure 14 Intact convergence with miosis in the patient shown in Figure 8 with paralysis of upward gaze due to pineal region tumor. The pupils were areflexic to light.

this important sign.[34] (Fig. 16). A beat or short burst of convergent-retraction nystagmus is observed each time the patient makes an upward saccade to refocus on the target. This method will evoke convergent-retraction nystagmus in virtually all patients with paralysis of upward gaze from a lesion of the rostrodorsal midbrain, but the sign will be overlooked unless the optokinetic test is performed.

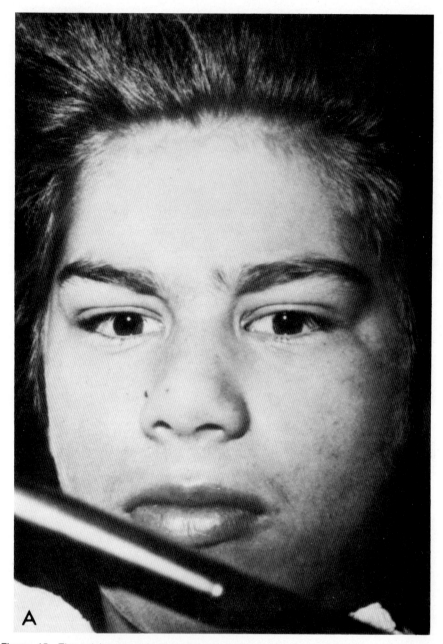

Figure 15 The sylvian aqueduct syndrome with paresis of upward gaze and spasmodic convergent-retraction nystagmus. **A.** Gaze straight ahead. **B.** Attempted upward gaze. Note here that the pupils did not constrict despite the marked convergent movement on attempted upward gaze. (Reproduced by permission from Walsh, FB, Hoyt WF: Clinical Neuro-ophthalmology. Williams and Wilkins, Baltimore, 1969).

The pathophysiology of the ocular movement disorder manifest as convergent-retraction nystagmus is not known. Gay and coworkers[4] concluded from EMG data that the normal reciprocal innervation of agonist and antagonist

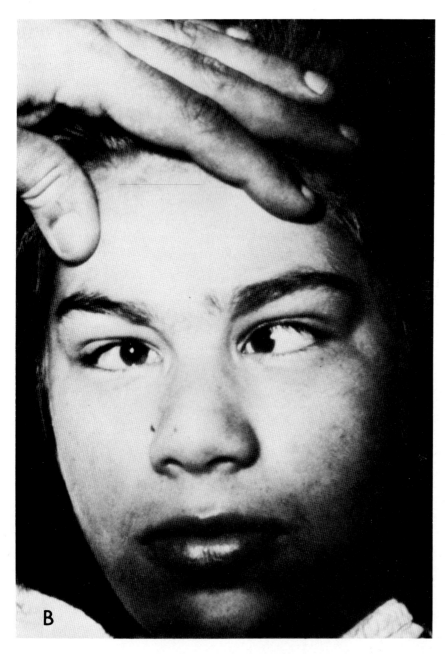

B

eye muscles was impaired. They published convincing evidence that simultaneous bursts of muscle activity occurred in all muscles innervated by the oculomotor and abducens nerves. When they examined EMG recordings from the medial and lateral rectus muscles, they found that bursts of *coinnervation* of the two muscles consisted of rapidly alternating reciprocal excitation and inhibition. From these data they suggested that convergent-retraction movements result from a disturbed pattern of innervation in antagonist muscles,

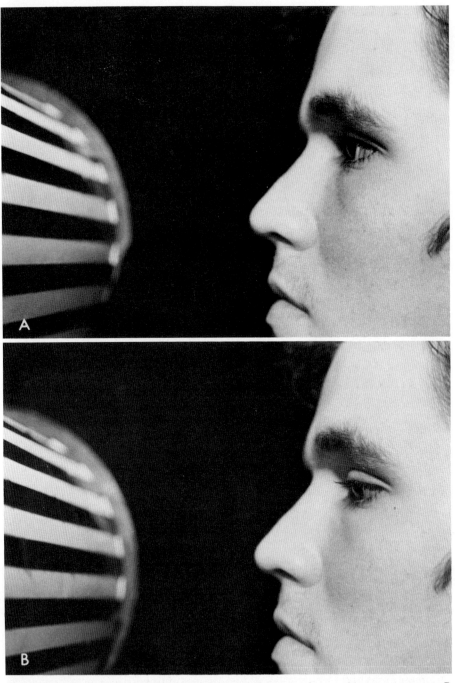

Figure 16 Convergent-retraction nystagmus. **A.** Position of eye without nystagmus. **B.** Position of eye during bout of retraction nystagmus. The stimulus was a downward rotating optokinetic drum. The patient had an epidermoid cyst of the pineal region (Case 13).

causing them to contract simultaneously. Recently, at the University of California in San Francisco, Ochs and coworkers,[5] using infrared photocell recording techniques, analyzed the amplitude-velocity relationship of convergent eye movements in a patient with typical signs and symptoms of pretectal involvement. The patient's eyes made multiple convergent jerks following every attempt to look upward, following some lateral shifts of fixation, and on occasions without apparent attempts to shift fixation. Plots of amplitudes and peak velocities of multiple convergent jerks showed typical amplitude-velocity relationships of saccades (Fig. 17). Thus, the convergent or opposed movements of the two eyes were caused by organized bursts of activity in cells of the oculomotor nuclei, with reciprocally linked inhibitory activity in the abducens nuclei. The fact that the convergent movements, as measured by Ochs and coworkers, exceeded the velocities of normal vergence movements by a factor of 10 proves that the opposed movements cannot be explained by phasic activity in the control system for vergence. Instead the movements represent perverted activity in the central control system responsible for rapid parallel eye movements, ie., saccades. Apparently the excitatory-inhibitory coupling between motonerons in the medial rectus subnucleus and the abducens nucleus is not interrupted by lesions that cause convergent-retraction nystagmus.

Why a lesion in the region of the aqueduct of Sylvius results in perverted activity in the pontine saccade generators has yet to be explained.

Lid Retraction and Other Lid Phenomena

Another eye sign in the patients with pinealomas, albeit a rare one, is pathologic retraction of the eyelids. This supranuclear type of lid retraction, Collier's sign, also termed the *posterior fossa stare,* is usually associated with paresis of upward gaze, which may be limited to a defect of voluntary movement.[48, 26] Lid retraction is symmetric and sustained so long as the patient directs his eyes straight ahead or slightly upward[26] (Fig. 18). It may be accompanied by excess or infrequent blinking. With downward gaze, the tone of the levator decreases smoothly and the lids follow the eye downward in a normal fashion. When the patient again looks up, lid retraction appears as the eyes reach the horizontal. Continued upward elevation of the eyes to look up increases the disparity between the position of the upper lids and the eyes. Walsh and Hoyt[26] have observed retraction of the upper lids in a boy with a pinealoma when his gaze was directed downward. This is unusual. Collier's sign has been attributed to compression of levator inhibitory fibers in the posterior commissure.[48, 49*]

A clinical photograph and measurements of the palpebral fissure in the primary position are valuable to document Collier's sign.

Skew Deviation and Paralysis of Oculomotor Nerves

Skew deviation, a nonparalytic vertical divergence of supranuclear origin or secondary to vestibulo-ocular disruption, may occur in patients with pineal

---

* A reversible Collier's sign is especially noteworthy in infants with hydrocephalus.

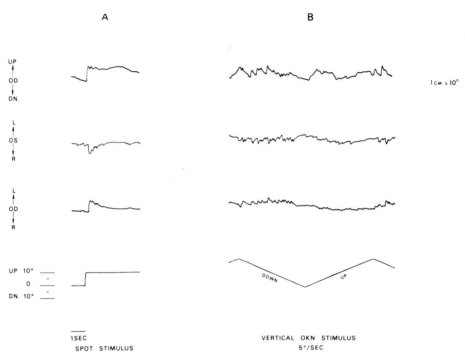

Figure 17   Sylvian aqueduct syndrome. Infrared photocell recording of horizontal eye movements. Electro-oculogram of vertical eye movement of the right eye (top trace). **A.** Convergent-nystagmus evoked by an intentional upward saccade. Note the rapid bilateral convergent movement and a slower divergence. **B.** Downward moving OKN stimuli evoke rapid irregular oscillatory eye movements and a convergence of the optical axes. Upward moving OKN stimuli no response. The disconjugate bilateral adductions have normal saccadic velocities. (Reproduced by permission from Ochs, A. L., Damico, D., Hoyt, W. F., et al.: Convergence saccades in a patient with convergent-retraction nystagmus (Parinaud's syndrome). Personal communication, 1976).

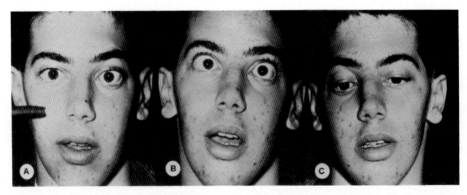

Figure 18   Collier's sign, or lid retraction with a lesion of the upper midbrain. **A.** This patient has a distinct stare (lid retraction) when looking straight ahead. **B.** Lid movement on attempted upward gaze is normal but the patient is unable to elevate his eyes. **C.** The "lid retraction" disappears on downward gaze. (Reproduced by permission from Walsh, F. B., Hoyt, W. F.: Clinical Neuro-Ophthalmology. Williams and Wilkins, Baltimore, 1969).

region tumors and cause vertical diplopia. Sanders and Bird[2] noted a skew in 3 of 10 cases of pinealoma and Cogan[43] a left hypotropia in one of his. Intermittent, periodic, alternating skew has also been observed.[50] Skew may be concomitant, laterally concomitant, or nonconcomitant and may mimic a single vertical muscle paresis.[51] The sign implicates brainstem or cerebellar disease but otherwise has no specific localizing value. Keane[52] has suggested that skew deviation may result from injury to the otolith ocular pathways, which are known to extend diffusely through the brainstem and are thought to influence vertical eye movements.

Nuclear oculomotor pareses may develop in pineal region tumors with invasion of the neoplasm ventral to the aqueduct. A unilateral third nerve nuclear lesion might be expected to involve most of the oculomotor muscles on the ipsilateral side, the superior rectus on the contralateral side, and both levators. Poppen and Marino[23] report a single case. Bilateral paralysis of the fourth nerves was the outstanding sign of a pineal tumor in Jaensch's case verified by autopsy.[53] The nucleus of the sixth nerve has almost no chance of suffering direct damage by tumor. But, since acute elevation of intracranial pressure is a prominent feature in pineal region tumors due to aqueduct stenosis, sixth nerve palsies, often bilateral, are frequently encountered. Posner and Horrax[22] report an incidence of 25%.

> Interested readers are referred to Gay et al.[25] to review the clinical examination of a patient with diplopia and the red-glass test for confirmation of a paretic ocular muscle.

Papilledema

In spite of the slow growth of pineal region tumors their location above the aqueduct of Sylvius leads to the obstruction and hydrocephalus. Thus, papilledema, which was present in 56% of patients in one series,[22] is an important sign,[22, 54, 55] but tells nothing about the diagnosis when it occurs by itself.

Early findings in papilledema are venous engorgement with loss of spontaneous venous pulsation.[56] There is also engorgement of fine vessels with hyperemia of the disc and edematous clouding of the nerve fiber layer, particularly at the disc margins. Hemorrhage in the nerve fiber layer, cotton wool spots, or microinfarcts may develop. Initially, there is no visual loss in papilledema beyond enlargement of the blind spot.

In pineal region tumors the disc swelling, when present, is usually similar in appearance in the two eyes and often severe, of the order of three to four diopters. With chronic papilledema, the central field is always depressed and often scotomatous and the peripheral visual field constricted. Visual obscurations may occur and secondary optic atrophy supervene. The visual loss in secondary atrophy follows ischemic involution of papilledema and is primarily nasal. This is accompanied by both a loss of disc color and elevation as well as arteriolar narrowing, often with some glial sheathing. To arrest this process the intracranial pressure should be lowered as soon as possible.

To facilitate detection of progressive change in the severity or resolution of papilledema, measure, in diopters, with the ophthalmoscope the degree of optic disc swelling in each eye. When available, obtain serial fundus photographs.

B. Ectopic Pinealomas

Chapter 6 is devoted to a detailed discussion of ectopic pinealomas. But, this chapter, primarily concerned with the neuro-ophthalmic and neurologic manifestations of pineal region tumors, would be incomplete without mention of this entity.

In 1961 dysgerminomas in the anterior third ventricle were recognized by Kageyama and Belsky[57] as the cause of a distinctive clinical syndrome. In some cases there is both pineal area and anterior third ventricle involvement. Anterior third ventricle tumors, although isolated, were usually interpreted as seedings from a primary tumor of the pineal body.[58–62] Nevertheless, in 14 of the 50 cases reviewed by Kageyama and Belsky, and in two additional cases of their own, the optic chiasma-infundibular region was the apparent site of origin of the tumor.

Ectopic pinealomas produce a variable triad of symptoms: diabetes insipidus, hypopituitarism, and visual field defects.

Visual Field Defects

In the series of suprasellar dysgerminomas reported by Simson et al.[62] all 11 patients had visual field defects; 9 of the 11 had diabetes insipidus but only 3 had the triad of symptoms. Importantly, visual field loss due to involvement of anterior optic pathways is the reason most patients seek medical attention. The visual field defect may be slowly progressive, rapid, monocular, bitemporal, or homonymous due to compression and/or infiltration of the optic nerves, chiasm, and optic tracts. It may be associated with primary optic atrophy. Usually, however, the fields have the bitemporal signature of chiasmal involvement. Since these often occur during the prepubertal years, it is worth mentioning that accurate perimetric data can be obtained in young children in direct proportion to the skill and patience of the examiner. In light of this, any child presenting with diabetes insipidus and normal growth should be examined regularly for the appearance of chiasmal signs and should be considered a candidate for *ectopic* pinealoma until computerized axial tomography (CT scan) or pneumoencephalography (PEG), or both, exclude this possibility.

Pneumoencephalography with polytomography is still the most valuable study in the investigation of suprasellar tumors, since tomograms show the anatomic detail of the chiasm and anterior third ventricle better than the CT scan. Frequently, the PEG reveals neoplasm behind the optic chiasm and irregularly indenting the floor of the third ventricle. In these cases cerebrospinal fluid pressure is normal but the protein content is often elevated and there is a lymphocytic pleocytosis.*

---

* The spinal fluid is normal in patients with optic and hypothalamic gliomas.

Surgery is required to decompress visual pathways and to confirm the diagnosis prior to definitive treatment. At craniotomy the dysgerminoma is usually situated beneath and behind the optic chiasm which it displaces and infiltrates. Tumor tends to spread along the optic nerves.[63, 64] It may also infiltrate the optic tracts and extend into the infundibulum and hypothalamus. In the absence of severe optic atrophy, postoperative recovery of vision may however be remarkably good.[58]

Optic Atrophy

Unilateral or bilateral primary atrophy of the optic nerve is a frequent sign in suprasellar dysgerminoma patients. Pathologic changes in the optic nerve may be caused either by compression of the anterior visual system by tumor or by infiltration. In previous reports optic atrophy has most often been caused by tumor infiltration into optic nerve fibers.[63, 64]

Oculomotor Dysfunction

Paralysis of the third, fourth, and sixth oculomotor nerves occurs infrequently in cases of ectopic pinealoma. One example of ophthalmoplegia involving all the ocular motor nerves in the right eye was an 11-year-old boy experiencing *passing out spells*, headache, and emesis. Neuroradiologic studies revealed an enlarged sella and a suprasellar mass. Craniotomy disclosed a dysgerminoma extending into the sella and right cavernous sinus.[62] In a second case of unilateral ophthalmoplegia, reported in the same series, the patient complained of unilateral eye pain, diplopia, and intermittent emesis. He died shortly after a suprasellar dysgerminoma was exercised.

Combined Pineal Region and Anterior Third Ventricle Tumors

The major clinical consideration in a patient with the characteristic signs and symptoms of a discrete pineal region tumor is to determine whether a second tumor focus is present in the anterior third ventricle (and vice versa). A coexisting tumor in the suprasellar region can indicate a multicentric origin or suggest that an implant of neoplastic cells shed into the spinal fluid is growing as a metastasis in the infundibulum. Cytologic examination of the spinal fluid might provide the answer in such cases because exfoliated cells should drift down into the spinal subarachnoid space.

"Seeding" throughout the Neuraxis

Seeding throughout the neuraxis is well known with tumors originating in the pineal region. Several reports document dissemination of dysgerminoma into the spinal subarachnoid space.[65–68] The longest interval between an apparent cure of the pineal region tumor, with radiation therapy or local treatment, and spinal recurrence was 5 years. The metastases may be only 1.0 to 2.0 mm in diameter, are typically at the level of the conus medullaris, and initially do not usually cause symptoms. The subsequent neurologic picture is fairly typical of a lesion in the conus medullaris and cauda equina, with involvement of multiple nerve roots one after the other. But, several spinal metastases may occur and compress the cord at different levels.

A confusing clinical picture suggesting meningoencephalitis is reported with a highly malignant form of germ cell tumor of the pineal region, called the *endodermal sinus tumor*.[68] At necropsy there was leptomeningeal involvement with multiple intracranial and spinal tumors. (Extradural spread of pinealomas only occurs when there has been a preceding craniotomy.)

Of the pineal tumors of glial origin that metastasize to the spinal cord, the ependymoma is the most common, but it is very unusual for an ependymoma of the pineal area to metastasize to the suprasellar region by invading along the hypothalamus.

The Massachusetts General Hospital Patient Series

Twenty-two cases of tumor of the pineal region, the infundibular region, or both, occurring between 1971 and 1976, were reviewed for this study (Tables 1–3). Thirteen cases came from the author's personal files and the remainder from the files of Dr. Paul Chapman and members of the Department of Neurosurgery at the Massachusetts General Hospital. They constitute a separate group to the series of 53 cases already reported from this hospital.[69]

The tumors were verified pathologically in 16 cases; in 12 from tissue obtained at craniotomy, in 1 from biopsy of a spinal tumor (case 16), in 2 from cytologic examination of spinal fluid (cases 8 and 22), and in 1 from finding at necropsy (case 1). The tumors were classified cytologically as dysgerminoma in 7 cases, pinealoblastoma in 1, astrocytoma in 6, epidermoid cyst in 1, and an endodermal sinus tumor in 1.[68] In 2 of the 7 cases of dysgerminoma the tumor was suprasellar (cases 18 and 20). In 3 of the 7, separate tumors occupied the pineal and infundibular area (cases 8, 16, and 22).

In the 6 nonpathologically verified cases, diagnosis of dysgerminoma was presumed in 5 and an astrocytoma in 1 (case 14) from clinical and neuroradiologic data, including computerized axial tomography. It should be emphasized that less than half of our cases had the tumor cell character of what was once called *pinealoma*. Further, the high incidence of glial and other nonpineal gland tumors underscores the need for tissue diagnosis.

The average age at presentation was 19 years, the range being 6 to 35 years. The ratio of males to females was 15:7, reflecting the predominance reported by others.

The duration of symptoms before tumor diagnosis varied from 6 weeks to 4 years. The average was approximately 7 months. In this series the tumor presented in three ways: with visual problems, headache, or with neuroendocrine disorders.

Ocular Symptoms and Signs

Table 1 shows the overall frequency of visual symptomatology including a symptom of acquired myopia with disordered accommodation[2, 26] (cases 6 and 11), and unexplained vertical diplopia and blurred vision of various origin.

The frequency of upward gaze palsy, convergent-retraction nystagmus and pupillary areflexia to light stimulation is also evident in Table 1. The disjunctive ocular dyskinesia or *nystagmus* always consisted of convergent-retraction movements of the eyes. In one instance (case 13) convergent-retraction nystagmus occurred paroxysmally in the primary position of gaze and followed horizontal saccades, causing serious reading problems. In 2 patients (cases 5 and 13) every blink was accompanied by a burst of convergent-retraction jerking of the eyes.

Neurologic Symptoms and Signs

Table 2 shows the frequency of neurologic symptomatology. Headache was the major complaint in 15 of the 22 patients and the reason for seeking medical attention in 12. Papilledema was associated with headache in 10 patients. Seizures, not usually present in pineal region tumors, occurred in 4 of the cases with severe hydrocephalus, all of whom required a shunt procedure.

Symptoms and signs of spinal cord involvement occurred in only 2 patients 20 and 24 months after the diagnosis of an endodermal sinus tumor (case 19) and dysgerminoma (case 16).

The cerebrospinal (CSF) was examined in 12 patients and found to be abnormal in 9, with elevation of the spinal fluid protein and a lymphocyte pleocytosis. A cytologic examination for malignant cells was performed in 13 patients and was positive in 3 for cells consistent with a diagnosis of dysgerminoma (Table 3).

A CT scan was positive in all 14 patients in whom the test was performed (Table 3). The scan indicated a single mass lesion in the pineal region in 9

Table 2. Neurologic Symptoms and Signs and Spinal Fluid Changes in 22 Cases of Pinealoma

		No. of patients
Symptoms	Headache	15
	Seizures	4
Late	Leg weakness	2 ⸱
Signs	Papilledema	10
Late	Spinal cord signs	2
Spinal Fluid Protein (mg%)	40–59	1
	60–79	2
	80–99	3
	100–119	2
	over 120	1
Sugar (mg%)	Less than 40	9
Mononuclear cells	0–5	2
	6–9	1
	10–19	2
	20–29	2
	30–100	1
	Over 400	1
Xanthochromia	One plus	3
Gold sol	Insuffient data	
Malignant cells	Positive	3

Table 3. Massachusetts General Hospital Series of 22 Patients with Pineal Region Tumors and Ectopic Pinealomas

Case	Age	Presenting Symptoms	Pupils Size	Reaction Light	Reaction Acc	Gaze palsy Upward	Gaze palsy Downward	Pareses Converg	Nerve 3,4,6th	Skew	Attempted upward gaze	Elicited with OKN drum	Acuity	Fields	Papilled Diopters	Optic atrophy	Normal	PR	SS	Metastasis	Protein (mg%)	Lymph/mm	Cytology	CT scan	Pathology
1.	15	Headache	Dilated	Poor	Good	+	0	0	0	Alternating	+	NT	20/50 20/30	Constricted	4			+			NT	NT	NT	NT	Dysgerminoma
2.	6	Headache Seizures	Dilated	Poor	NT	+	0	NT	0	nating 0	0	NT	NT	NT	2			+			NT	NT	NT	NT	Dysgerminoma
3.	13	Headache Diplopia	Dilated	Poor	Good	+	0	0	0	Comitant	0	+	20/20 OU	Full	2			+			94	2	0	+	Dysgerminoma
4.	33	Headache	Dilated	Fixed		+	0	0	Bilat 4th	0	+	+	20/30 OU	Full	2			+			80	16	0	NT	Astrocytoma grade III
5.	16	Headache	6 mm	Poor	Good	+	0	0	0	0	+	+	Myopic	Full		+		+			62	5	0	+	Astrocytoma grade III
6.	13	Headache Blurred vision Diplopia Diabetes insipidus	Anisocoria 4, 7 mm	Poor	Good	+ Bell's reflex absent	0	0	0	Alternating	0	+	20/30 OU	Full			+	+			Normal			+	Dysgerminoma
7.	27	Headache	8 mm	Poor	Good	+	0	+	0	0	+	+	20/20	Full			+	+			80	20	0	+	Dysgerminoma, presumed
8.	18	Headache Seizures Blurred vision	6 mm	OD Amaurotic OS Poor	Good OS	0	0	0	0	0	0	NT	20/400 OD 20/20 OS	Central & bitemporal defect	3				+		Not recorded		+	+	Dysgerminoma
9.	16	Diplopia	6 mm	Poor	Good	Upbeat Nystag.	0	0	0	R. hyper	0	+	20/25 20/30	Full			+	+			Normal		0 0	+ +	Dysgerminoma, pre-

44

Table 3 Continued

Case	Age	Presenting Symptoms	Pupils Size	Reaction Light	Reaction Acc	Gaze palsy Upward	Gaze palsy Downward	Pareses Converg	Nerve 3, 4, 6th	Skew	Attempted upward gaze	Elicited with OKN drum	Vision Acuity	Vision Fields	Papilled Diopters	Optic atrophy	Normal (Fundi)	PR	SS	Metastasis	Protein (mg%)	Lymph/mm	Cytology	CT scan	Pathology
10.	15	Headache		Poor	Good	0	0	0	0	0	0	NT	20/200	Constricted	3			+			NT	NT	NT	NT	Dyserminoma, presumed
11.	30	Headache Diplopia	Aniso-coria	Poor	Good	0	0	+	0	Alternating	0	+	My-opic	NT			+	+			NT	NT	NT	NT	Astrocytoma
12.	15	Headache		Normal		0	0	0	R.6th	0	0	NT	20/40	NT				+			NT	NT	NT	NT	Astrocytoma
13.	21	Headache Difficulty reading	6 mm	Poor	Good	+	0	+	0	0	+ (Spontaneous and hor gaz)	+	20/30 20/25	Full		+		+			NT			+	Epidermoid cyst
14.	18	Diplopia	7 mm	Poor	Good	+	0	0	0	0	+	+	My-opic	Full				+			Normal			+	Astrocytoma, presumed
15.	35	Headache Diplopia		Poor	Good	+	0	0	0	0	+	NT									Normal	Normal		NT	Pinealoblastoma
16.	30	Diabetes insipidus Loss libido		Poor	Good (Amaurotic)	0	0	0	Bilat 6th	0	0	0	20/30 20/40 Progressed to blindness	Bitemp hemianopia Progressed to blindness					+	Spinal	69	20	+	+	Dyserminoma
17.	22	Headache Diplopia	3 mm	Normal		+	0	0	0	0	0	NT	20/30	Constricted	3			+			100	2	0	+	Astrocytoma, grade 1
18.	15	Growth failure Amenorrhea Poor vision Diabetes insipidus	3 mm	Normal		0	0	0	0	0	0	0	20/25 20/30	Bitemp hemianopia			+				44	19	0	+	Dyserminoma

Table 3—Continued

Case	Age	Presenting Symptoms	Pupils Size	Reaction Light	Reaction Acc	Gaze palsy Upward	Gaze palsy Downward	Pareses Converg	Nerve 3, 4, 6th	Skew	Attempted upward gaze	Elicited with OKN drum	Acuity	Fields	Papilled Diopters	Optic atrophy	Normal	PR	SS	Metastasis	Protein (mg%)	Lymph/mm	Cytology	CT scan	Pathology
19.	12	Diabetes insipidus Lethargy	Anisocoria 3 mm, 7 mm	Normal		0	0	0	6th N palsy	0	0	NT	20/30	NT	3			+	Leptomeninges	Spinal	137	400	0	+	Endodermal sinus tumor
20.	8	Growth failure Diabetes insipidus		Normal		0	0	0	0	0	0	NT	20/25	NT	3				+		Not recorded		0	+	Dysgerminoma
21.	25	Headache	3 mm	Normal		0	0	0	0	0	0	NT	20/20	Full			+	+	+		Normal			NT	Astrocytoma grade I
22.	22	Blurred vision Diabetes insipidus		Amaurotic		0	0	0	0	0	0	0	20/400 OD CF 1' OS	Bitemp defect				+	+		100	96	+	+	Dysgerminoma

+ Present
0 Absent
NT Not tested
PR Pineal region
SS Suprasellar

46

patients, a single suprasellar tumor in 2 patients (cases 18 and 20), and both a pineal region tumor and an ectopic suprasellar mass in 3 patients (cases 8, 16, and 22). The details of other neuroradiologic findings are not discussed since Chapter 4 reviews this topic.

Neuroendocrine Disorders

Six of the 22 patients had diabetes insipidus associated, in some cases, with other signs and symptoms of hypopituitarism. One patient had primary hypothyroidism.[68] Interestingly, in another child with a suprasellar dysgerminoma anorexia nervosa was the initial diagnosis (case 18). A similar case has been reported.[70] Chapter 3 is devoted to a full discussion of the neuroendocrine effects of pineal region and ectopic pinealomas.

Illustrative Cases

Clinical data from all 11 patients are given in Table 3. Selected cases are reported in detail.

> *Case 18.* A 15-year-old girl weighing 90 lb, and 4 ft 11 inches tall, looked younger than her stated age. She attended an adolescent clinic because of primary amenorrhea. Anorexia nervosa was diagnosed. No endocrine studies were done. Six months later she noted impaired vision in the temporal field of the right eye and diabetes insipidus. On examination visual acuity was 20/40, read left-hand letters only right eye (OD) 20/25, read right-hand letters only left eye (OS). Visual fields were full to a large target, but the isopter charted for the smallest dimmest target the patient could see showed bitemporal hemianopic scotoma (Fig. 19). The pupils, ocular motility, OKN responses, and fundus examination were normal. A CT scan revealed a solid suprasellar mass. A PEG showed a mass irregularly indenting the floor of the third ventricle. No abnormality was noted in the region of the pineal. The CSF protein was 44 mg % and contained 19 lymphocytes. The cytologic examination for malignant cells was

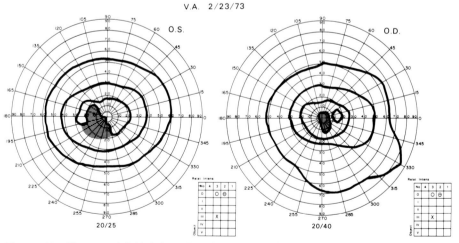

V.A. 2/23/73

Figure 19 Bitemporal field defects in a 15 year old girl with a suprasellar dysgerminoma producing difficulty in reading. The child carried an initial diagnosis of anorexia nervosa (case 18).

negative. A transfrontal craniotomy was performed and a suprasellar dysgerminoma excised. There was no recovery of the visual field defect. Whole brain irradiation, 4,000 rads, was given plus an additional boost of 650 rads to the anterior third ventricle. The patient, under treatment for diabetes insipidus, is doing well 3 years following treatment. The visual impairment has not progressed.

Comment. This case illustrates the importance of recognizing growth failure.[70] School children are now required by law to be weighed and measured every year. The data should be graphed so that aberrant growth patterns can be more easily detected. Visual impairment was a late manifestation.

Case 22. A 22-year-old man noted blurred vision in the left eye. An ophthalmologist found the visual acuity OD 20/20, OS 20/30 + 1, and a "generalized constriction" of the field OS. The left disc appeared pale. Ten months later vision had deteriorated to 20/200 OS and diabetes insipidus developed. A suprasellar mass was shown on PEG. The spinal fluid contained 56 mg % protein and 11 lymphocytes. Craniotomy was performed but no obvious tumor identified. "The pituitary stalk appeared larger than usual, with distended veins along the anterior surface." A biopsy was taken from the hypothalamic region and showed *focal hypoplasia.* Five months later rapid visual loss occurred in the right eye, and he was referred for a second opinion. On examination, visual acuity 20/400 OD, counting fingers at 1.0 foot OS, amaurotic pupils, dense bitemporal field defect and severe bilateral optic atrophy. Ocular motility was intact with no convergent-retraction nystagmus. PEG and CT scan revealed two mass lesions, one in the suprasellar area indenting the anterior third ventricle and one in the posterior third ventricle in the pineal region. Dysgerminoma cells were identified in the spinal fluid and grown in tissue culture. The patient received radiotherapy to the whole neuroaxis but without improvement in vision. The patient, under treatment for diabetes insipidus, remains well 1 year later.

Comment. This case illustrates the value of cytologic examination of the spinal fluid in patients with unexplained optic atrophy and radiologic evidence of a suprasellar mass.

Infratentorial-Supracerebellar Operation

The oculomotor effects of the infratentorial supracerebellar operation for pineal region tumor were recorded in 5 cases. The operative approach, described first in 1926 by Krause,[71] has been adopted recently by Suzuki and Iwabuchi,[72] and by Stein.[73] Such a route to the pineal region has the advantage of avoiding the vein of Galen and the internal cerebral veins, which usually lie in relation to the dorsal or lateral aspects of the tumor. It also permits the surgeon to open the third ventricle into the quadrageminal cistern and establish the flow of spinal fluid when the aqueduct is blocked. An internal shunt from the third ventricle into the upper cervical subarachnoid space can be inserted. While this approach affords a good view into the superior regions of the third ventricle towards the foramen of Monro, it does not permit clear visualization downward. Thus, if tumor extends inferiorly toward the midbrain it cannot be readily seen without considerable retraction of the superior vermis and tectal plate. To overcome this disadvantage a parasagittal approach to the pineal gland area is still favored by some surgeons, since this technique facilitates inspection of the posterior inferior regions of the third ventricle.

Mass lesions in the pineal region were excised by this technique in 5 patients (cases 5, 6, 13, 17, and 25) in the Massachusetts General Hospital series. Four of the patients were observed to have tumor invading the pretectal-collicular area of the brainstem. In 1, symptomatic with headache but with no neurologic or ocular signs, an astrocytoma was partially removed (case 25). She remains well 6 months later. A second patient with astrocytoma, papilledema, and paresis of upward gaze made a full recovery following operation. Her improvement was attributed to decompression of the aqueduct (case 17). A 4-month-old sylvian aqueduct syndrome resolved 2 months after surgery for a dysgerminoma (case 6).

Illustrative Cases

Case 5. The first case seen by the author, pre- and postoperative, following partial excision of a grade III astrocytoma by the infratentorial approach was a 16-year-old girl with a known pineal region tumor for 4 years. A shunt had been inserted 2 years previously. Preoperative examination showed pupil areflexia to light, paresis of upward gaze, paralysis of convergence, and convergent-retraction nystagmus. In the immediate postoperative period the patient showed a striking lack of all random eye movements. She sat staring straight ahead. The normal movements of fixation and following were completely abolished, so that she failed to move either head or eye to seek or follow objects of interest brought into view. She blinked infrequently but there was no lid retraction. She conversed normally with her examiners. During the following 6 months the patient slowly improved, and horizontal and downward eye movements recovered. Paralysis of upward gaze with convergent-retraction nystagmus, paralysis of convergence, and pupil areflexia to light persisted. When last seen 4 years later, in January 1977, the patient was well. Signs of the sylvian aqueduct syndrome remained unchanged.

Comment. Myers[74] described similar visual behavior, or lack of it, in cats after stereotactic lesions in the superior collicus, ventral periaqueductal gray matter, and the ventral tegmentum. The patient's immediate postoperative signs were attributed to the effects of traction on the pretectal region.

Case 13. A 26-year-old man with a known posterior third ventricle mass since age 11 was referred for treatment. He had prominent signs of a periaqueductal lesion with paresis of upward gaze, convergent-retraction nystagmus, and pupils areflexic to light stimuli. He had previously received irradiation therapy to the pineal region at age 12 and a shunt procedure was performed at age 24. Prior to suboccipital craniotomy, the CT scan, without contrast, revealed a mass lesion in the region of the pineal and splenium of the corpus callosum. The margins appeared partially calcified, the reading up to 400 units. The rest of the lesion had a very low absorption and in certain portions readings were down to minus 50 units. The findings were consistent with either a cystic dermoid or partially calcified lipoma of the splenium. A supracerebellar infratentorial approach was used to totally excise a noninvasive epidermoid cyst. Twelve hours after recovery from the anesthetic, he developed a left congruous homonymous hemianopia. A vertebral arteriogram showed no abnormality. The visual field defect recovered fully in the next 3 days. The ocular motility and pupil signs of the sylvian aqueduct syndrome remained unchanged. He returned to his home in Tennessee 1 month later and a follow-up visit to Boston has not yet taken place.

Comment. This case reemphasizes the need for a tissue diagnosis in patients with a mass demonstrated in the pineal region prior to radiation treatment. The value of computerized axial tomography to distinguish a cystic lesion from a solid tumor is especially noteworthy.

Neuroanatomy and Neurophysiology of Ocular Signs in Pineal Region Tumors

Anatomic Substrate of Vertical Gaze and Lid Control

While some advances have been made in the anatomy and physiology of eye movement control, the precise pathways by which impulses from the frontal and parieto-occipital cortex are conveyed to the oculomotor nuclei of extraocular muscles in the brainstem are unknown.

Area 8 is classically cited as the cortical motor area for generating the saccadic command signal.[75, 76] Stimulation of this area in the monkey produces saccadic eye movements.[77, 78] A brief unilateral stimulus produces a single contraversive horizontal saccade, simultaneous bilateral frontal cortical stimulation vertical saccadic movements.[78, 79] The simplistic view that all saccadic eye movements are initiated in the frontal eye fields is unlikely to be correct. First, because of the unnatural nature of electrical stimulation and second, and more importantly, because of findings from recent recordings from frontal cortex.[80, 81] In a study of normal activity of cells in area 8 in the alert monkey, Bizzi found no cells that fired prior to eye movement. Instead the cells fired during saccades. His findings, now corroborated by others, raise serious doubts that prefrontal *eye fields* are responsible for volitional saccades.[82] There has also been controversy regarding the neuroanatomy of frontomesencephalic and pontine pathways carrying eye movement signals, but now we cannot even define the function of this pathway if indeed it even exists. Experimental and clinical evidence suggests that the neural system subserving vertical gaze act bilaterally and that some of them descend in the anterior limb of each internal capsule, pass beneath the ventrolateral portion of the thalamic masses, through the region of the zona incerta and fields of Forel, into the ipsilateral reticular formation and subtectal nuclei of the rostral midbrain.[83, 84]

The deep subcortical systems for smooth pursuit movements appear closely associated with those for saccades. The occipitomesencephalic fibers from the peristriate cortex pass medial to the optic radiations (internal saggital stratum) through the retrolenticular zone in the posterior limb of the internal capsule, through the pulvinar, and to the pretectal reticular formation. Horizontal pursuit involvements appear clinically to be regulated by the ipsilateral occipital cortex but again this simplistic conception has no factual support from the laboratory. Vertical pursuit is bilaterally regulated at all levels above the rostral mesencephalon.[79]

Bilaterally the descending fiber systems mediating control of vertical pursuit are spatially and probably synaptically associated with the fronto-mesencephalic fiber subsystems in the pretectal region of the midbrain. This convergence of corticobulbar oculomotor fiber systems in the pretectum does not imply functional unity for vertical saccades and pursuit systems. Lesions in the rostral midbrain can differentially involve upward and downward gaze. For the system controlling upward gaze, there is a fiber decussation in the posterior commissure, but for the system controlling downward gaze, there is no apparent decussation. Electrical stimulation experiments in monkeys and cats suggest that upward ocular deviations occur more frequently from rostrodorsal stimulation in the midbrain, while downward deviations occur mostly from ventrocaudal stimulation of the midbrain.[79, 85, 86]

Certain accessory nuclei related to the oculomotor nucleus of the midbrain seem to be essential for control of vertical eye movement. These nuclei are the paired interstitial nuclei of Cajal, the nuclei of Darkschewitsch, and the nuclei of the posterior commissure.

The interstitial nucleus of Cajal lies outside of the central periaqueductal gray matter, among and lateral to the fibers of the medial longitudinal fasciculus (MLF) in the rostral midbrain. Descending fibers from the interstitial nucleus of Cajal run in the MLF to project to the trochlear nuclei, to the caudal portion of the vestibular nuclei, and to the other lower brainstem nuclei.[87] Discrete unilateral lesions of the interstitial nucleus of Cajal produce primarily disturbances of head posture. This nucleus appears to be important for integration of tilting movements of the head in a frontal plane with conjugate vertical and rotatory movements of the eyes.[88, 89]

The nucleus of Darkschewitsch lies inside the ventrolateral border of the central periaqueductal gray matter, dorsal and lateral to the nuclear columns of the third nerve nuclear complex. Rostrally this nucleus begins in the gray matter near the site where the fasciculus retroflexus traverses the red nucleus. It is dorsal to the interstitial nucleus of Cajal and to the MLF and does not give rise to any fibers that enter the MLF.[87] Conclusions concerning the precise function of the nucleus of Darkschewitsch are difficult to draw since discrete lesions have not been confined to this nucleus in experimental studies.[90] Fibers of the interstitial nucleus of Cajal, which cross in the posterior commissure, and variable amounts of the lateral periaqueductal gray matter have been concomitantly involved. The affected monkeys have shown bilateral eyelid retraction and impairment of vertical eye movements, particularly those associated with upward gaze. Some investigators contend that neither the nuclei of Cajal and of Darkschewitsch are essential for control of vertical eye movement.[91] Instead they claim that fiber systems in the posterior commissure are indispensable for control of vertical gaze.

The nuclei of the posterior commissure lie outside the central periaqueductal gray matter, intimately associated with fibers of the posterior commissure. No fibers from nuclei of the posterior commissure descend in the MLF. Bilateral lesions of ventrally crossing fibers in the posterior commissure in the monkey produce paresis of upward gaze, lid retraction and convergent-retraction nystagmus.

While the role of accessory oculomotor nuclei in vertical gaze remains enigmatic and the fact that no locale has been identified as the integrator of upward eye movements, the pretectal area of the midbrain can be considered the functional upward gaze *center* in the same way that we consider the pontine paramedian reticular formation to be the pontine center for horizontal gaze. Opinion is firm that the superior colliculi do not play an indispensable role in the activation of vertical eye movements.[91, 92] But, this in no way excludes some significant contribution of the superior colliculi to precision in vertical eye movement control.

From the finding that lesions in the pretectum may affect upward gaze alone and that lesions in the anterior part of the mesencephalon may produce isolated paralysis of downward gaze, it seems that there is some sort of separation of eye movement in various directions somewhere in the midbrain. Components for downward gaze lie ventrocaudally to the fasciculus retroflexus just ventral to the aqueduct and medial-dorsal to the red nucleus. In three autopsy studies in patients with discrete paralysis of vertical downward gaze, the eye signs were due to bilateral *butterfly* lesions situated beneath the aqueduct in the anterior part of the mesencephalon.[93-95] In two of these cases[93, 94] bilateral involvement extended from the thalamus medial to the red

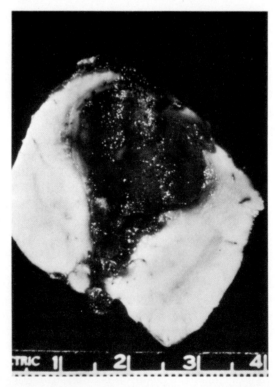

Figure 20 Rostral midbrain section at the level of the superior colliculi showing extensive dysgerminoma blocking the aqueduct of Sylvius and destroying the posterior commissure, dorsal tegmentum and peri-aqueductal region. The patient had paralysis of upward gaze, areflexic pupillary light reflexes and convergent-retraction nystagmus.

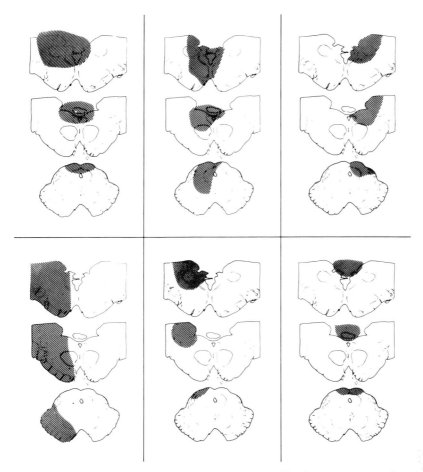

Figure 21   Top left: tumor of bilateral pretectum, dorsal midbrain tegmentum and posterior commissure; paralysis of upward gaze. **Top center:** tumor of bilateral pretectum, dorsal and ventral tegmentum and posterior commissure; paralysis of up and down gaze. **Top right:** tumor involving unilateral pretectum, tectum and posterior commissure; paralysis of upward gaze. **Bottom left:** unilateral tumor of midbrain without pretectum or posterior commissure involvement; no paralysis of gaze. **Bottom center:** compression of midbrain and posterior commissure without invasion; no paralysis of gaze. **Bottom right:** tumor from corpus callosum involving tectum but not pretectum; no paralysis of gaze. (Reproduced by permission from Christoff, N., A clinicopathologic study of vertical eye movements. *Arch. Neurol.* **31**, 1–8 (1974).)

nuclei, through the fasciculus retroflexus, and back into the central gray with destruction of the nuclei of Darkschewitsch and the interstitial nucleus of Cajal.

Anatomic Pathways for Convergence

The anatomic pathways for vergence movements are not known. They may descend, possibly from the peristriate region to the pretectal area of the midbrain, with the occipitomesencephalic pathways. For some time authors

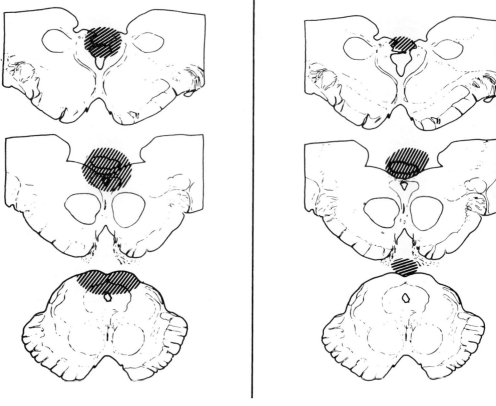

Figure 22   Left: Invasion of pretectum and posterior commissure by pineal tumor; paralysis of upward gaze. **Right:** Compression of the pretectum by pineal tumor; no paralysis of gaze. (Reproduced by permission from Christoff, N.: A clinicopathologic study of vertical eye movements. *Arch. Neurol.* **31**, 1–8 (1974).)

regarded the central nucleus of Perlia as the cell group concerned with convergence.[96] But, from the work of Warwich and others the very existence of a nucleus of Perlia seems fictitious.[97, 98]

Pathologic Changes from Pineal Region Tumors

Clinical studies, no matter how carefully done, have limited value in determining anatomic components of a motor control system. Clinicopathologic studies of tumors is also the least likely to yield information on topology[20, 40–42] (Fig. 20, case 1). The data from discrete vascular lesions in the rostral midbrain have therefore been reviewed.[49, 93–95, 99, 100] The vascular necropsy cases are also important in the light of work by Nashold and Gills who have produced typical pretectal syndromes in 8 patients with intractable pain, treated by unilateral electrocoagulation of the midbrain tegmentum adjacent to the posterior commissure.[101]

We have also noted a clinicopathologic study of vascular and tumor patients by Christoff. He included 27 patients with paralysis of vertical gaze,

6 of whom had pinealomas, compared with 34 patients in whom there were lesions in similar locations but without vertical gaze paralysis[102] (Figs. 21 and 22).

From these data we conclude: bilateral lesions of the pretectal nuclei, a single midline posterior commissural lesion, or a unilateral midbrain tegmental lesion involving a substantial number of crossing fibers in the posterior commissure can produce the sylvian aqueduct syndrome. Isolated destruction of the superior colliculi does not produce obvious clinical alterations of eye movements. Unilateral involvement of posterior commissure fibers can produce Collier's sign.[49,101] Bilateral anterior mesencephalic lesions rostral to the oculomotor nuclei produce paralysis of downward gaze.[93-95] Insufficient ocular observations have hampered the clinicopathologic correlation of Bell's reflex.

Acknowledgment

This study was supported in part by Grant No. NS11551 awarded by the National Institute of Neurological and Communicative Disorders and Stroke, D.H.E.W., and in part by a grant from Fight for Sight, Inc., New York City.

References

1. Daroff, R. B., and Hoyt, W. F., Supranuclear disorders of ocular control systems in man: Clinical, anatomical and physiological correlations, *The Control of Eye Movements*. Edited by P. Bach-y-Rita, and C. C. Collins. Academic Press, New York, 1971, pp 175-235.
2. Sanders, M. D., and Bird, A. C., Supranuclear abnormalities of the vertical ocular motor system. *Trans. Ophthalmol. Soc. U.K.* **90**, 433-450 (1970).
3. Esslen, E., and Papst, W., Die Bedeutung den Elektromyographie für die Analyse von Motilitätsstorungen der Augen. *Bibl. Ophthalmol. Suppl.* **57**, 1-168 (1961).
4. Gay, A. J., Brodkey, J., and Miller, J. E., Convergence retraction nystagmus. *Arch. Ophthalmol,* **70**, 456-461 (1963).
5. Ochs, A. L., Damico, D., Hoyt, W. F., and Stark, L., Convergence saccades in a patient with convergence-retraction nystagmus (Parinaud's syndrome). Personal communication (1976).
6. Collins, C. C., O'Meara, D., and Scott, A. B., Muscle tension during unrestrained human eye movements. *J. Physiol.* **245**, 351-369 (1975).
7. Daroff, R. B., and Troost, B. T., Supranuclear disorders of eye movements, *Clinical Ophthalmology,* vol. 2. Edited by T. D. Duane. Harper and Row, Hagerstown, Md., 1976.
8. Cogan, D. G., *Neurology of the Ocular Muscles,* Second edition. C. C Thomas, Springfield, 1956.
9. Schwartz, G. A., and Rosner, A. A., Displacement and herniation of the hippocampal gyrus through the incisura tentorii. A clinicopathologic study. *Arch. Neurol. Psychiat.* 46, 297-321 (1941).
10. Lerner, M. A., Kosary, I. Z., and Cohen, B. E., Parinaud's syndrome in aqueduct stenosis: its mechanism and ventriculographic features. *Br. J. Radiol.* **42**, 310-312 (1969).
11. Shallat, R. F., Pawl, R. P., and Jerva, M. J., Significance of upward gaze palsy (Parinaud's syndrome) in hydrocephalus due to shunt malfunction. *J. Neurosurg.* **38**, 717-721, 1973.
12. Swash, M., Periaqueductal dysfunction (the Sylvian aqueduct syndrome): a sign of hydrocephalus? *J. Neurol. Neurosurg. Psychiatry* **37**, 21-26 (1974).

13. Chattha, A. S., and Delong, G. R., Sylvian aqueduct syndrome as a sign of acute obstructive hydrocephalus in children. *J. Neurol. Neurosurg. Psychiatry* **38**, 288–296 (1975).
14. Bielschowsky, A., Lecture on motor anomalies of the eyes. III. Paralysis of conjugate ocular movements of the eye. *Arch. Ophthalmol.* **13**, 569–583 (1935).
15. Man, H. X., A propos d'un cas de paralysie supra-nucleaire unilaterale des muscles elevateurs. *Bull. Soc. Ophthalmol. Fr.* **67**, 400–405 (1967).
16. Jampel, R. S., and Fells, P., Monocular elevation paresis caused by a central nervous system lesion. *Arch. Ophthalmol.* **80**, 45–57 (1968).
17. Lessell, S., Supranuclear paralysis of monocular elevation. *Neurology* **25**, 1134–1136 (1975).
18. Chamberlain, W., Restriction in upward gaze with advancing age. *Am. J. Ophthalmol.* **71**, 341–346 (1971).
19. Hoyt, W. F., Personal communication (1976).
20. Gowers, W. R., Case of intracranial disease with optic neuritis and paralysis of the upward movement of both eyes. *Trans. Ophthalmol. Soc. U.K.* **1**, 117–119 (1881).
21. Parinaud, H., Paralysie des mouvements associés des yeux. *Arch. Neurol.* **5**, 145–172 (1883).
22. Posner, M., and Horrax, G., Eye signs in pineal tumors. *J. Neurosurg.* **3**, 15–24 (1946).
23. Poppen, J. L. and Marino, R., Pinealomas and tumors of the posterior portion of the third ventricle. *J. Neurosurg.* **28**, 357–364 (1968).
24. Tod, P. A., Porter, A. J., and Jamieson, K. G., Pineal tumors. *Am. J. Roentgenol. Radium Ther. Nucl. Med.* **120**, 19–26 (1974).
25. Gay, A. J., Newman, N. M., Keltner, J. L., and Stroud, M. H., *Eye Movement Disorders.* C. W. Mosby, St. Louis (1974).
26. Walsh, F. B., and Hoyt, W. F., *Clinical Neuro-ophthalmology.* Williams and Wilkins, Baltimore (1969).
27. Seybold, M. E., Yoss, R. E., Hollenhorst, R. W., and Moyer, N. J., Pupillary abnormalities associated with tumors of the pineal region. *Neurology* **21**, 232–237 (1971).
28. Lowenstein, O., Alternating contraction anisocoria: Pupillary syndrome of anterior midbrain. *Arch. Neurol.* **72**, 742–757 (1954).
29. Wilson, S. A., Ectopia pupillae in certain mesencephalic lesions. *Brain* **29**, 524–536 (1906).
30. Selhorst, J. B., Hoyt, W. F., Feinsod, M., and Hosobuchi, Y., Midbrain corectopia. *Arch. Neurol.* **33**, 193–195 (1976).
31. Parinaud, H., Paralysis of the movement of convergence of the eyes. *Brain* **9**, 330–341 (1886).
32. Kestenbaum, A., *Clinical Methods of Neuro-ophthalmologic Examination.* Grune and Stratton, New York, 1946, p. 214.
33. Kornblueth, W., Transient abolition of the pupillary reaction in the presence of intact convergence and accommodation to convergence, and normal pupillary reaction to accommodation in a case of tumor of the pineal gland. *Am. J. Ophthalmol.* **35**, 1815–1820 (1952).
34. Smith, J. L., Zieper, I., Gay, A. J., and Cogan, D. G., Nystagmus retractorius. *Arch. Ophthalmol.* **62**, 864–867 (1959).
35. Cogan, D. G., and Freese, C. G., Jr., Spasm of the near reflex. *Arch. Ophthalmol.* **54**, 752–759 (1955).
36. Griffin, J. F., Wray, S. H., and Anderson, D. P., Misdiagnosis of spasm of the near reflex. *Neurol.* **26**, 1018–1020 (1976).
37. Herman, P., Convergence spasm. *Mt. Sinai J. Med. N.Y.*, 1976, in press.
38. Nieden, A., Ein Fall von bilateraler Associations-Parese der Rect. superior et oblique inferiores, mit Auftreten von klonischen Zuckungen in den übrigen Augen-Muskelgruppen. *Centralbl. f. Prakt. Augenheilk.* p. 209–213, 1880. Cited by Sanders, M. D., and Bird, A. C., Supranuclear abnormalities of the vertical ocular motor system. *Trans. Ophthalmol. Soc. U.K.* **90**, 433–450 (1970).

39. Koerber, H. L., Ueber drei Fälle von Retraktionsbewegung des Bulbus. *Ophthalmol. Klin.* **7**, 65–67 (1903).
40. Salus, R., Über erworbene Retraktionsbewegungen der Augen. *Arch. Kinderkeilk* **47**, 61–76 (1910).
41. Elschnig, A., Nystagmus retractorius, ein cerebrales Herdsymptom. *Med. Klin.* **9**, 8–11 (1913).
42. deManchy, S. J. R., Rhythmical convergence spasm of the eyes in a case of tumor of the pineal gland. *Brain* **46**, 176–188 (1923).
43. Cogan, D. G., Convergence nystagmus. *Arch. Ophthalmol.* **62**, 295–298 (1959).
44. Segarra, J. M., and Ojemann, R. J., Convergence nystagmus. *Neurology* **11**, 883–893 (1961).
45. Barany, E., Verein für Psychiatrie and Neurologie in Wien. *Wien. Klin. Wochenschr.* **26**, 480–482 (1913).
46. Christoff, N., Anderson, P. J., and Bender, M. B., Convergence and retractory nystagmus. *Trans. Am. Neurol. Assoc.* **85**, 29–32 (1960).
47. Atkin, A., and Bender, M. B., "Lightning eye movements" (ocular myoclonus). *J. Neurol. Sci.* **1**, 2–12 (1964).
48. Collier, J., Nuclear ophthalmoplegia, with special reference to retraction of the lids and ptosis and to lesions of the posterior commissure. *Brain* **50**, 488–489 (1927).
49. Hatcher, M. A., Jr., and Klintworth, G. K., The sylvian aqueduct syndrome. A clinico-pathologic study. *Arch. Neurol.* **15**, 215–222 (1966).
50. Cogan, D. G., and Wray, S. H., Unpublished data.
51. Smith, J. L., David, N. J., and Klintworth, G., Skew deviation. *Neurology* **14**, 96–105 (1964).
52. Keane, J. R., Ocular skew deviation. Analysis of 100 cases. *Arch. Neurol.,* **32**, 185–190 (1975).
53. Jaensch, P. A., Doppelseitige Trochlearisparese als einzige Motilitätssörung bei Zir-beldrüsentumor. *Z. Augenheilk* **75**, 58–68 (1931). Cited by Walsh, F. B. and Hoyt, W. F., *Clinical Neuro-ophthalmology.* Williams and Wilkins, Baltimore (1969).
54. Kunicki, A., Operative experiences in 8 cases of pineal tumor. *J. Neurosurg.* **17**, 815–823 (1960).
55. Russell, W. O., and Sachs, E., Pinealoma. A clinicopathologic study of seven cases with a review of the literature. *Arch. Pathol.* **35**, 869–888 (1943).
56. Kahn, E. A., and Cherry, G. R., The clinical importance of spontaneous retinal venous pulsations. *Univ. Mich. Med. Bull.* **16**, 305–308 (1950).
57. Kageyama, N., and Belsky, R., Ectopic pinealoma in the chiasma region. *Neurology* **11**, 318–327 (1961).
58. Baker, G. S., and Rucker, C. W., Metastatic pinealoma involving the optic chiasm. *J. Neurosurg.* **1**, 377–378 (1950).
59. Dayan, A. D., Marshall, A. H. E., Miller, A. A., Pick, F. J., and Rankin, N. E., Atypical teratomas of the pineal and hypothalamus. *J. Pathol. Bact.* **92**, 1–28 (1966).
60. Rand, R. W., and Lemmen, L. J., Tumours of the posterior portion of the third ventricle. *J. Neurosurg.* **10**, 1–18 (1953).
61. Stringer, S. W., Diabetes insipidus associated with pinealoma transplant in the tuber cinereum. *Yale J. Biol.* **6**, 375–383 (1933–34).
62. Simson, L. R., Lampe, I., and Abell, M. R., Suprasellar germinomas. *Cancer* **22**, 533–544 (1968).
63. Sano, K., Nagai, M., Mayanagi, Y., and Basugi, N., Ectopic pinealoma in the chiasmal region in childhood. *Dev. Med. Child. Neurol.* **10**, 258–259 (1968).
64. Kageyama, N., Ectopic pinealoma in the region of the optic chiasm. Report of five cases. *J. Neurosurg.* **35**, 755–759 (1971).
65. Baggenstoss, A. H., and Love, J. G., Pinealomas. *Arch. Neurol. Psychiatr.* **41**, 1187–1206 (1939).
66. Fowler, F. D., Alexander, E., Jr., and Davis, C. H., Jr., Pinealoma with metastases in the central nervous system: A rationale of treatment. *J. Neurosurg.* **13**, 271–288 (1956).

67. Case Records of Massachusetts General Hospital. *N. Engl. J. Med.* **284**, 1427–1434 (1971).
68. Case Records of Massachusetts General Hospital. *N. Engl. J. Med.* **291**, 837–843 (1974).
69. DeGirolami, U., and Schmidek, H., Clinicopathological study of 53 tumors of the pineal region. *J. Neurosurg.* **39**, 455–462 (1973).
70. Clinicopathologic conference: a case of anorexia. *Br. Med. J.* **2**, 156–161 (1973).
71. Krause, F., Operative Freilegung der Vierhügel, nebst Beobachtungen über Hirndruck und Dekompression. *Zbl. Chir.* **53**, 2812–2819 (1926).
72. Suzuki, J., and Iwabuchi, T., Surgical removal of pineal tumors (pinealomas and teratomas): experience in a series of 19 cases. *J. Neurosurg.* **23**, 565–571 (1965).
73. Stein, B., The infratentorial supracerebellar approach to pineal lesions. *J. Neurosurg.* **35**, 197–202 (1971).
74. Myers, R. E., Visual deficits after lesions of brain stem tegmentum in cats. *Arch. Neurol.* **11**, 73–90 (1900).
75. Holmes, G., The cerebral integration of the ocular movements. *Br. Med. J.* **2**, 107–112 (1938).
76. Ferrier, D., The localization of function in the brain. *Proc. R. Soc. B.* **22**, 229–232 (1874).
77. Krieger, H. P., Wagman, I. H., and Bender, M. B., Change in state of consciousness and patterns of eye movements. *J. Neurophysiol.* **21**, 224–230 (1958).
78. Robinson, D., and Fuchs, A., Eye movements evoked by stimulation of frontal eye fields. *J. Neurophysiol.* **32**, 637–648 (1969).
79. Bender, M. B., Comments on the physiology and pathology of eye movements in the vertical plane. *J. Nerv. Ment. Dis.* **130**, 456–466 (1960).
80. Bizzi, E., Discharge of frontal eye field neurons during saccadic and following eye movements in unanesthetized monkeys. *Exp. Brain Res.* **6**, 69–80 (1968).
81. Bizzi, E., and Scheller, P. H., Single unit activity in the frontal eye fields of unanesthetized monkeys during eye and head movements. *Exp. Brain Res.* **10**, 151–158 (1970).
82. Mohler, C., Goldberg, M. E., and Wurtz, R. H., Visual receptive fields of frontal eye neurons. *Brain Res.* **61**, 385–389 (1973).
83. Brucher, J. M., The frontal eye field of the monkey. *Int. J. Neurol.* **5**, 262–281 (1966).
84. Bender, M. B., and Shanzer, S., Oculomotor pathways defined by electric stimulation and lesions in the brainstem of monkey. *The Oculomotor system.* Edited by M. B. Bender. Harper and Row, New York, 1964, pp 81–140.
85. Spiegel, E. A., and Scala, N. P., Ocular disturbances associated with experimental lesions of the mesencephalic gray matter. *Arch. Ophthalmol.* **18**, 614–630 (1937).
86. Bender, M. B., Pathways mediating vertical eye movements. *Trans. Am. Neurol. Assoc.* **84**, 159–161 (1959).
87. Pompeiano, O., and Walberg, F., Descending connections to the vestibular nuclei. An experimental study in the cat. *J. Comp. Neurol.* **108**, 465–502 (1957).
88. Hyde, J. E., and Toczek, S., Functional relation of interstitial nucleus to rotatory movements evoked from zona incerta stimulation. *J. Neurophysiol.* **25**, 455–466 (1962).
89. Hyde, J. E., and Eason, R. G., Characteristics of ocular movements evoked by stimulation of brain stem of cat. *J. Neurophysiol.* **22**, 666–678 (1959).
90. Carpenter, M. B., Central ocular motor pathways, *The Control of Eye Movements.* Edited by P. Bach-y-Rita, and C. C. Collins. Academic Press, New York, 1971, pp 67–103.
91. Pasik, P., Pasik, T., and Bender, M. B., The pretectal syndrome in monkeys. I. Disturbances of gaze and body posture. *Brain* **92**, 521–534 (1969).
92. Balthasar, K., Gliomas of the quadrigeminal plate and eye movements. *Ophthalmologica* **155**, 249–270 (1968).
93. Thomas, A., Schaefer, H., and Bertrand, I., Paralysie de l'abaissement du regard, paralysie des inférogyres, hypertonie des superogyres et des releveurs des paupières. *Rev. Neurol.* **2**, 535–542 (1933).

94. Jacobs, L., Anderson, P. J., and Bender, M. B., The lesions producing paralysis of downward but not upward gaze. *Arch. Neurol.* **28,** 319–323 (1973).
95. Cogan, D. G., Paralysis of down-gaze. *Arch. Ophthalmol.* **91,** 192–199 (1974).
96. Knies, M., Ueber die centralen Störungen de willkurlichen Augenmuskein. *Arch. f. Augenheilk.* **23,** 19–51 (1891).
97. Warwick, R., The so called nucleus of convergence. *Brain* **78,** 92–114 (1955).
98. Clarke, W. E. L., The mammalian oculomotor nucleus. *J. Anat.* **60,** 426–488 (1926).
99. Környey, S., Blickstörungen bei vasculären Herden des mesodiencephalen Übergangsgebietes. *Arch. Psychiat. Nervenkr.* **198,** 535–543 (1959).
100. Molnar, L., Die lokaldiagnostiche Bedeutung der vertikalen Blicklähmung. *Arch. Psychiat. Nervenkr.* **198,** 523–534 (1959).
101. Nashold, B. S., Jr., and Gillis, J. P., Jr., Ocular signs from brain stimulation and lesions. *Arch. Ophthalmol.* **77,** 609–618 (1967).
102. Christoff, N., A clinicopathologic study of vertical eye movements. *Arch. Neurol.* **31,** 1–8 (1974).

CHAPTER THREE
Endocrine Dysfunction in Patients with Tumors of the Pineal Region

Lloyd Axelrod   Boston, Massachusetts

ENDOCRINE DYSFUNCTION IS such a frequent concomitant of tumors of the pineal region that the endocrine status of all patients with these neoplasms must be assessed regularly. Although precocious puberty in males is the most widely known endocrine abnormality associated with pineal region tumors, it is merely one of several endocrine disturbances that beset patients with such neoplasms. These tumors are not infrequently associated with isolated hypogonadism, with diabetes insipidus, and with anterior pituitary insufficiency. Although abnormalities of sexual maturation are readily apparent, diabetes insipidus and anterior pituitary insufficiency may be less obvious but more of a threat to the survival of the patient. The purpose of this chapter is to summarize current concepts of the physiology of the pineal gland in mammals, to review endocrine and metabolic disorders associated with tumors of the pineal gland, and to suggest an approach to the evaluation of endocrine function in patients with suspected or proved neoplasms of the pineal region.

Physiology of the Pineal Gland

Notable advances in our understanding of the function of the pineal gland have occurred in recent years as a result of achievements in several separate areas of investigation; reviews of these developments are available.[1-10]

Until recently, tradition had stigmatized the pineal gland as a vestigial remnant of the parietal eye and a subject worthy of philosophers (as the seat of the soul), which served only to permit the recognition of midline shifts on x-rays of the skull. A more contemporary view must account for the following:

1. A striking functional evolution of the pineal has occurred.[11] In fish and

Assistant Professor of Medicine, Massachusetts General Hospital, Boston, Massachusetts

amphibians the principal pineal cell is a neurosensory photoreceptor cell, very similar in structure to the retina of the eye. However, in reptiles and birds pineal photosensory function is gradually lost, and in mammals the pinealocyte is a secretory cell (Table 4).

2. The mammalian pineal contains and can synthesize an indole called melatonin. It is virtually the only organ in the body that can do so, because it contains the enzyme responsible for the last step in the synthesis of this molecule, hydroxyindole-O-methyl transferase.

3. The mammalian pineal has acquired innervation from the sympathetic nervous system. The input to the pineal cells appears to be mediated by norepinephrine released from the sympathetic nerves. Norepinephrine increases the synthesis of melatonin by stimulating a β-adrenergic receptor on the membrane of the pineal cell. This results in the activation of adenylate cyclase within the cell, and the synthesis of cyclic adenosine monophosphate. The latter increases the activity of an enzyme, N-acetyltransferase, which converts serotonin (a precursor of melatonin) to N-acetylserotonin (an intermediate in the pathway of melatonin synthesis). This appears to be the critical step in the control of pineal melatonin synthesis. Both darkness and the setting of an internal biologic clock are necessary for the nocturnal increase in N-acetyltransferase activity.[12]

4. Although the mammalian pineal gland lacks neurosensory function and cannot respond directly to light stimulation, this organ responds indirectly to environmental light by a pathway that begins at the eye and the optic nerves, passes through the brainstem and spinal cord, and then concludes with postganglionic sympathetic fibers that originate in the superior cervical ganglia and terminate at the parenchymal cells of the pineal (Fig. 23). This organ is inhibited by light and stimulated (or released from inhibition) by darkness.

5. The pineal gland produces a substance (or substances) capable of inhibiting gonadal growth and function. This conclusion is based on numerous animal studies of the effect of pinealectomy on gonadal size, weight, or growth. In their extensive review of the world literature, Kitay and Altschule[13] found that gonadal hypertrophy was observed in the majority of such studies. Some contradictory results obtained in early studies may have been due to failure to appreciate and control the effects of light on pineal and gonadal function.[2] Studies taking such factors into account have recently provided more consistent evidence that the pineal gland inhibits the gonads

Table 4. Pineal Physiology in Experimental Animals

1. The pineal exerts an antigonadotropic effect, which may be mediated by melatonin or another substance (or substances).
2. Light inhibits (and darkness augments) pineal function.
3. The response to light involves a pathway that includes the eyes, optic nerves, brainstem, spinal cord, and postganglionic sympathetic fibers, which originate in the superior cervical ganglia and terminate at the parenchymal cells of the pineal.
4. Blindness or darkness results in decreased gonadal size.
5. This system may be of adaptive value to species with seasonal reproductive rhythms by insuring that birth of offspring occurs in the spring.

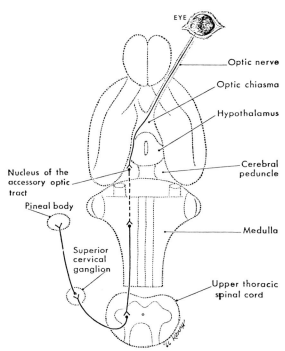

EYE

Optic nerve

Optic chiasma

Hypothalamus

Cerebral peduncle

Nucleus of the accessory optic tract

Pineal body

Medulla

Superior cervical ganglion

Upper thoracic spinal cord

Figure 23 Neural pathway between retina and pineal gland in mammals. Photoreceptors in eye respond to light by generating impulses transmitted by the optic nerve. Most of these impulses travel to brain centers associated with vision. A small fraction of the impulses diverges from the main visual pathway and travels along the inferior accessory optic tract, which leads to the central hypothalamic neurons involved in the regulation of the sympathetic system. The pathway then descends via the spinal cord to preganglionic neurons, which supply the superior cervical ganglia; postganglionic neurons ascend to the pineal where they act by regulating the neurotransmitter norepinephrine. (Reprinted, by permission, from Wurtman, R. J., Axelrod, J., Kelly, D. E., The Pineal. Academic Press, New York, 1968.

in animals of both sexes, but only to a moderate degree in most species.[2] It is not yet possible to designate the pineal substance or substances that mediate this antigonadal effect. Melatonin, the first compound to be considered for this role, is still the leading contender.[8, 10] This substance inhibits the synthesis and release of luteinizing hormone, apparently through an action on brain structures (ie., the median eminence and midbrain reticular substances) controlling the pituitary gland.[14] But other substances of pineal origin exert antigonadal effects, including compounds related in structure to melatonin (such as 5-methoxytryptophol and 5-hydroxytryptophol) and a compound (or compounds) unrelated in structure and thought to be a polypeptide (or polypeptides).[8-10]

A contemporary scheme of pineal physiology would then represent this organ as one indirectly subject to environmental light. By a pathway involving the eyes, the central nervous system, and the sympathetic nervous system light inhibits (and darkness augments) pineal function. The pineal exerts an antigonadotropic effect that may be mediated by melatonin or another substance (or substances) that acts to suppress the synthesis and release of luteinizing hormone. Decreased gonadal size would then result from blindness or darkness or from interruption of the neural pathway, which transmits light to the pineal gland (as by obliteration of the superior cervical ganglia).

Of what value is it to an organism to have a photosensitive organ that regulates gonadal function? The adaptive value may be the regulation of seasonal reproductive rhythms to insure that the birth and nurturing of offspring occur during the spring, when conditions for survival are optimal. There is evidence that during seasons of decreased light there is increased pineal antigonadotropic activity, and that during seasons of increased light, the pineal is suppressed and the gonads regenerate.[5, 9]

It is hazardous to draw conclusions about the physiology of the human pineal gland, and specifically about the abnormalities of sexual maturation associated with pineal tumors in man, from studies in experimental animals. Although the above formulation is founded on a large body of experimental observations in many species, there are relatively few data on pineal physiology in man. Recent studies demonstrate the existence of diurnal rhythms of melatonin in normal human subjects.[15-17] A nocturnal rise in plasma levels of melatonin in human volunteers is detectable by both bioassay[15, 16] and radioimmunoassay.[16] Similarly, the melatonin content of urine samples collected from human volunteers between 11 PM and 7 AM is higher than that of samples collected between 7 AM and 3 PM, or between 3 PM and 11 PM, when measured by bioassay.[17] Because humans do not have seasonal reproductive rhythms, it is unlikely that these variations in plasma levels and urinary excretion rates of melatonin have the same physiologic significance in humans as in experimental animals. There is evidence that environmental light does not have the same effect on reproductive function in humans as it does in experimental animals. Because the antigonadotropic effects of the pineal in animals are most apparent in darkness, one might expect that blindness would produce a delay in the age of menarche. In fact, the opposite occurs. Blindness is associated with an earlier onset of menarche than that observed in girls with normal vision.[18] Kitay and Altschule[13] found reports of 9 patients with primary hypoplasia of the pineal gland: 8 had sexual precocity, but 5 of these had pituitary lesions as well. They felt that the etiology of the sexual precocity could not be resolved from available data. They also found 6 reported cases of absence of the pineal gland: *hypogonadism* was present in 3. Although the physiologic significance of the pineal is unlikely to be the same in humans as in experimental animals, it will be of interest to learn about the regulation of melatonin secretion as further use is made of bioassays and immunoassays of this substance.

Endocrine Manifestations of Tumors of the Pineal Region

The endocrine manifestations of tumors of the pineal region include abnormalities of sexual maturation, diabetes insipidus, and anterior pituitary insufficiency.

Abnormalities of Sexual Maturation

Abnormalities of sexual maturation, particularly precocious puberty but also delayed sexual maturation, are among the most striking manifestations of pineal tumors. Perhaps for this reason, and also because of the possible physiologic implications of such abnormalities, they have until recently overshadowed other endocrine consequences of these tumors.

The reported incidence of *sexual precocity* among patients with pineal tumors varies markedly (Table 5). Kitay and Altschule[13] found 46 reported cases in patients with verified pineal tumors (all males under 17 years of age) among 606 patients with such neoplasms. Since they found reports of 178 pineal tumors in patients from 1 to 16 years old (145 in boys), they calculated an overall incidence of precocity in this age group of 26%; and an incidence in males only in this age range of 32%. David analyzed 108 reported cases of verified pineal tumors in children; 34% had precocious puberty, including 43% of the males, and 50% of males with a *teratoma*.[19] However, a lower incidence has been encountered in other series, ranging from 11% of 19 cases[20] to 0% of 12 patients (ref. 21, cited in 22) and 0% of 65 patients, 14 of whom were less than 15 years old.[23] The higher figures in the series of cases collected from the

Table 5.   Precocious Puberty and Tumors of the Pineal Region

A. Frequency of Precocious Puberty in Patients with Tumors of the Pineal Region

Source	Frequency	Frequency in subpopulations
Kitay and Altschule,[13] review of literature (1954)	8% of total cases (46 of 606 patients of all ages)	26% of all patients from 1 to 16 yr old 32% of male patients from 1 to 16 yr old
Ringertz et al.,[23] series from the Neurosurgical Clinic of the Serafimer Lasarettet, Stockholm 1954	0% of total cases (65 patients of all ages, 14 younger than 15 yr)	
David,[19] review of literature 1957	34% of total cases (37 of 108 children, 15 yr old or less)	43% of male children 50% of male children with "teratomas"
David,[20] series from Hôpital Debrousse, Lyon, 1963	11% of total cases (2 of 19 patients)	
Jallade,[21] thesis cited by Bovier-Lapierre et al.[22], 1966	0% of total cases (12 cases)	

B. Frequency of Pineal Region Tumors Among Children with Precocious Puberty

Source	All cases of precocious puberty	Cases of idiopathic precocious puberty	Cases of neurogenic precocious puberty (Cases of pineal tumors in boys)
Bing, Globus and Simon[24], 1938	474	380	94(21) 1938
Wilkins[25], 1965	70	606	96(22) 1965

Table adapted and revised from Bovier-Lapierre et al.[22]

literature may reflect a bias in favor of reporting cases associated with precocious puberty. Therefore, the lower figures may better reflect the true incidence of this abnormality. If the incidence of pineal region tumors in children with precocious puberty is examined, these neoplasms will be found to be an uncommon cause of this endocrine disturbance (Table 5). Precocious puberty associated with tumors of the pineal region occurs only in boys.[19, 22]

Three theories have been advanced to explain the association of precocious puberty with tumors of the pineal region[13, 20, 22] (Table 6):

1. The human pineal (like the animal counterparts described above) secretes a substance (or substances) with an antigonadotropic effect. Sexual precocity occurs when secretion of this substance is decreased as a result of destruction of pineal parenchymal cells by a tumor of nonparenchymal origin. (Isolated hypogonadism results from secretion of excessive quantities of this agent by a tumor of parenchymal origin.)

2. Tumors of the pineal region cause precocious puberty by an effect of the tumor mass. The expanding neoplasm compresses or destroys diencephalic areas that inhibit the sexual center of the median eminence, resulting in augmented secretion of gonadotropins and consequent precocity.

3. The tumor secretes an ectopic gonadotropin.

Until recently, only the first two theories received serious consideration. However, direct evidence for the secretion of an ectopic gonadotropin in a small number of patients with tumors of the pineal region puts the third theory on solid ground. It is worth considering the arguments for and against each hypothesis.

The idea that precocious puberty and isolated hypogonadism result, respectively, from decreases or increases in the secretion of a pineal antigonadotropic substance received strong impetus from the analysis of Kitay and Altschule.[13] They assumed that the functional status of the pineal, as a secretory organ, could be determined from the histology of the lesions, as reported in the literature. They asserted that since the normal pineal gland is composed of two types of cell, parenchymal and nonparenchymal, tumors of this gland could be similarly classified. They reasoned that if precocious puberty were explained by the pressure hypothesis, then this endocrine abnormality should be unrelated to the histologic structure of the pineal tumor. In their scheme, parenchymal tumors included lesions described as pinealomas, adenomas, and hypertrophy. Nonparenchymal tumors consisted primarily of mixed tumors and supporting tissue tumors, but included also a few cystomas, nerve-cell tumors, fibrolipomas, and germinomas. Of the 46

Table 6.   Possible Explanations for the Occurrence of Precocious Puberty in Boys with Tumors of the Pineal Region

1. The human pineal secretes an *antigonadotropic* substance. Sexual precocity occurs when secretion of this substance is *decreased* as a result of the destruction of pineal parenchymal cells by a tumor of nonparenchymal origin.
2. The expanding tumor produces loss of the inhibitory effects of the diencephalon on the median eminence resulting in augmented secretion of the gonadotropins and precocity.
3. The tumor secretes an ectopic gonadotropin.

reported cases of precocious puberty, which they analyzed, 10 were associated with parenchymal tumors and 36 with nonparenchymal tumors, although parenchymal and nonparenchymal lesions occurred with equal frequency in patients between 1 and 16 years of age. They concluded that since 78% of the cases of precocious puberty were associated with nonparenchymal tumors, the evidence favored the hypothesis that precocious puberty is due to destruction of normal parenchymal pineal tissue by nonparenchymal tumors, with decreased secretion of the pineal substance that inhibits gonadal development, and resultant precocity. David obtained similar results in a study of 108 verified pineal tumors in children. Of 71 children without precocity 42 had *pinealomas,* but of 37 with precocious puberty only 6 had *pinealomas.*[19, 20]

This hypothesis has no direct support, since levels of melatonin in body fluids have not been shown to correlate with the presence of precocity or isolated hypogonadism in patients with tumors of the pineal region. The availability of bioassay and radioimmunoassay methods for the measurement of melatonin in body fluids should facilitate study of this question. Clinical studies that demonstrate an association between precocious puberty and nonparenchymal tumors are not conclusive. They rest on the questionable assumption that the functional status of the pineal gland as a secretory organ can be determined from the histologic appearance of the lesions. They also assume that all reports of tumors of the pineal region use a single system of nomenclature and that all observers would agree on the classification of tumors of the pineal region, an obviously erroneous assumption in view of the existence of several systems of nomenclature for these neoplasms.

The second theory advanced to explain the association of precocious puberty with tumors of the pineal region states that the expanding neoplasm compresses or destroys diencephalic areas, with loss of diencephalic inhibitory effects on the median eminence and enhanced secretion of the gonadotropins from the anterior pituitary gland. Sexual precocity occurs in other organic diseases of the brain.[24-26] In children with diencephalic hamartomas precocity may be due to increased production of luteinizing hormone-releasing hormone; this substance has been found in high concentrations in the cerebrospinal fluid of 3 patients.[26] In other forms of cerebral disease (such as deformities, tumors, phacomatoses, chronic inflammatory processes, and hydrocephalus) it is thought that sexual precocity results from the premature activation of the sexual center of the median eminence, resulting from the abolition of inhibitory impulses from the posterior diencephalon.[26] In one review it was noted that in 21 cases of pineal tumor with precocious puberty, the neoplasm was not localized to the pineal region but had caused morphologic changes elsewhere in the brain, either by extension into such diencephalic areas as the quadrigeminal bodies, the thalamus, and the third ventricle or by obstruction of the aqueduct of Sylvius with resultant hydrocephalus. In 15 of the 21 cases precocious puberty was observed together with other abnormalities associated with hypothalamic dysfunction, including polydipsia, polyuria, polyphagia, somnolence, and obesity.[24] The authors of this study also pointed out that pineal tumors often produce such abnormalities of hypothalamic function without causing alterations in sexual maturation, and that alteration in sexual development may occur when the pineal is uninvolved. Accordingly, it was concluded that the hypothalamus, not the pineal body, is the probable seat of the disturbance that results in sexual precocity. It seems reasonable to conclude that in at least some patients with tumors of the pineal region precocious puberty is due to pressure effects of the tumor mass and loss of the inhibitory effects of the diencephalon on the median eminence of the hypothalamus.

The third explanation put forth to explain the presence of precocious puberty in patients with tumors of the pineal region is that there is ectopic production of a gonadotropic substance by the tumor. This theory is supported by direct evidence.[27-29] Cases have been described in which human chorionic gonadotropin (HCG), detected by specific radioimmunoassay techniques, was present at high levels in the serum of patients with precocious puberty and a tumor of the pineal region.[27-29] Only one such case has been reported in detail.[29] Another report described a girl with a germinoma of the anterior third ventricle but without sexual precocity, who had elevated levels of HCG detected by a specific radioimmunoassay.[30]

In view of the paucity of cases studied, it is not yet possible to determine whether the ectopic production of gonadotropin is frequently or infrequently the cause of sexual precocity associated with tumors of the pineal region. It is perhaps not unrelated that the most common group of tumors of the pineal region are those of germ-cell origin,[31] since germ-cell tumors arising elsewhere in the body (eg., the testis) are associated with the production of HCG.[32] One wonders how many of the *nonparenchymal* tumors reported to be associated with precocious puberty were in fact tumors of germ-cell origin producing HCG. Attribution of sexual precocity in patients with tumors of the pineal region to the ectopic production of HCG may account for the fact that sexual precocity in association with these lesions occurs only in males. Human chorionic gonadotropin resembles pituitary luteinizing hormone (LH) in that it has interstitial cell stimulating activity, but lacks significant follicle stimulating hormone (FSH) activity. The testis needs only stimulation of the interstitial cells to initiate sex steroid secretion, but the ovary needs both FSH and LH to elaborate estrogen.[33]

Isolated hypogonadism is also observed in association with tumors of the pineal region. In young children it is manifest by the delayed onset of puberty. In postpubertal children it is characterized by regression of secondary sex characteristics, with decreased breast size and disappearance of menstrual periods, and by decreased testicular size and loss of body hair. Kitay and Altschule[13] collected reports of 30 cases, in males from 6 to 35 years old. Although this complication occurs predominantly in males, it is also said to occur in females.[22]

The pathogenesis of isolated hypogonadism in patients with tumors of the pineal region is even less well understood than the pathogenesis of precocious puberty. Again, one can identify three possible explanations:

1. The production of excessive quantities of a substance with an antigonadotropic effect by tumors of parenchymal pineal origin; or

2. An effect of the tumor mass on hypothalamic function due to compression or destruction of cells that regulate the gonadotropic function of the anterior pituitary gland (such as cells that synthesize luteinizing hormone-releasing hormone); or

3. The nonspecific effect of systemic illness on hypothalamic-pituitary regulation of reproductive function.

Kitay and Altschule found that 20 of 30 reported cases of hypogonadism were associated with *parenchymal* tumors, while the remaining 10 had *nonparenchymal* lesions, a difference not statistically significant. They suggested that the association of parenchymal tumors with sexual retardation be examined further.[13] This theory receives indirect support from (a) the demonstration of high levels of the melatonin-forming enzyme, hydroxyindole-*O* methyl transferase in tumor tissue obtained at autopsy from a pinealoma arising in the anterior portion of the third ventricle of an 18-year-old girl;[34] (b) the demonstration of hydroxyindole-*O* methyl transferase, melatonin, and serotonin in a cutaneous metastasis removed from a 14-year-old boy with a mass in the pineal region, who had not entered puberty;[35] and (c) evidence, in experimental animals, that the normal pineal gland produces a substance (or substances) capable of inhibiting gonadal growth and function. Thus, there is only indirect support for the theory that when isolated hypogonadism occurs in association with tumors of the pineal region, it is due to the secretion of excessive quantities of a substance with an antigonadotropic effect by a parenchymal pineal tumor. The possibility that isolated hypogonadism is due to an effect of the tumor mass on the hypothalamus is more likely; in at least some cases it is a manifestation of the anterior pituitary insufficiency associated with tumors of the pineal region (see below). Certainly it is reasonable to suspect that hypogonadism in such patients may be due, in some cases, to the nonspecific effects of systemic illness; delayed onset of puberty and secondary amenorrhea both occur in association with a host of emotional and organic disorders. Clearly, such a diagnosis must be made after other possible causes of hypogonadism in the setting of a tumor of the pineal region are excluded. Since the presence of excessive amounts of melatonin (or other antigonadotropic substances) has not been excluded in such cases, and since the extent of the tumor mass is often poorly defined, the possibility that isolated hypogonadism is a nonspecific effect of stress is still conjectural.

In summary, the mechanism of sexual precocity in boys with tumors of the pineal region is not yet established. The hypothesis that precocious puberty is the result of destruction of pineal parenchymal cells by tumors of nonparenchymal origin, and a resultant decrease in the elaboration of an antigonadotropic substance or substances of pineal origin, is appealing because of the evidence for the existence of such agents in experimental animals; but this explanation lacks direct evidence. The hypothesis that such tumors cause precocity by an effect of the tumor mass receives support from the association of sexual precocity with other organic diseases of the brain, and from the fact that the majority of patients with precocious puberty and tumors of the pineal region also have other signs and symptoms of hypothalamic dysfunction. The concept that sexual precocity is due to the ectopic production of a gonadotropin by a tumor of the pineal region has been proven by the measurement of HCG by specific radioimmunoassay techniques in a small number of cases. It is not yet possible to state whether this is frequently or infrequently the mechanism of sexual precocity in patients with precocious puberty and tumors of the pineal region. It is of interest that the majority of tumors of the pineal region are of germ-cell origin, and that tumors of germ-cell origin arising elsewhere in the body are also associated with the ectopic production of gonadotropins. The occurrence of sexual precocity exclusively among male patients with tumors of the pineal region is consistent with the ectopic production of HCG by the neoplasm; HCG stimulates the interstitial cell of the testis to secrete androgens (with resultant sexual precocity) but does not contain FSH activity, which is also needed for enhanced estrogen synthesis by the ovary. The origin of isolated hypogonadism in patients with tumors of the pineal region is not known. There is no evidence that this abnormality occurs more frequently in patients with parenchymal tumors than in those with nonparenchymal tumors, nor that these patients have tumors that elaborate excessive quantities of melatonin or another pineal antigonadotropic substance. Isolated hypogonadism in some cases is likely to be due to an effect of the tumor mass on the hypothalamus; it may also occur as a nonspecific response to stress, a reasonable but unproven possibility.

Diabetes Insipidus

Diabetes insipidus is an important clinical manifestation of tumors of the pineal region; as a frequent concomitant of such tumors, its presence may herald the diagnosis and it can be treated.

Diabetes insipidus may be the most common endocrine abnormality associated with tumors of the pineal region (Table 7). The precise incidence cannot be determined for several reasons. In many reports the diagnosis is asserted on clinical grounds; strict criteria, utilizing plasma and urine osmolalities, are not employed.[36] In virtually all instances provocative tests are not reported, so that mild cases may have been overlooked. In some studies these deficiencies are due to the fact that the reports were published before the tests in question were available. In many cases, the illness of the patient appears to have precluded dehydration or other provocative tests of antidiuretic hormone reserve.

In determining the incidence of diabetes insipidus it is also necessary to distinguish between tumors of the pineal region and tumors that arise in the chiasmal region of the anterior third ventricle, the histologic appearance of which may be similar to that of tumors of the pineal region. These tumors of the chiasmal region have often been called *ectopic pinealomas,* an unfortunate term since, like tumors of the pineal region, they are often derived from tissues other than pineal parenchymal cells. The incidence of diabetes insipidus in patients with tumors of the pineal region is lower than that in patients with tumors of the chiasmal region.

When diabetes insipidus is associated with a tumor of the pineal region, it

Table 7. Occurrence of Diabetes Insipidus in Patients with Tumors of the Pineal Region or the Chiasmal Region

Source	Incidence of diabetes insipidus	Percent	Comment
Tumors of the pineal region (exceptions noted)			
Russell and Sachs[47]	1 of 7	14	Authors' series
(1943)	15 of 58	26	Review of literature, including authors' series
Horrax[37] (1947)	5 of 17	29	Author's series: 3 cases with tumors of pineal region, 1 with tumor of the pineal region involving hypothalamus and pituitary and 1 with "ectopic pinealoma" above the sella turcica.
Ringertz et al.[23] (1954)	4 of 65	6	Authors' series
Smith[45] (1961)	8 of 38	21	Author's series
	5 of 35 tumors of pineal region	14	
	3 of 3 cases of "ectopic pinealoma"	100	
Dayan et al.[48] (1966)	8 of 10	80	Authors' series: 6 cases with tumor of pineal region, 2 cases with pineal region free of tumor.
Tumors of the Chiasmal Region			
Rubin and Kramer[39] (1965)	8 of 8	100	Authors' series
	34 of 36	94	Review of literature, including authors' series.

is probably due to extension of the tumor from the pineal region to the hypothalamus and pituitary.[37, 38] There is pathologic evidence that this may occur by implantation of a discrete metastasis to the hypothalamus[38] or by extension of the tumor through the floor of the third ventricle to involve the hypothalamus and posterior pituitary gland.[37] Confusion may arise because such lesions may not be apparent by radiographic studies, such as a pneumoencephalogram or a ventriculogram. When diabetes insipidus is associated with a tumor of the chiasmal region that does not involve the pineal region it is likely that the endocrine disturbance is due to the location of the tumor mass in the neurohypophysis.[39] However, in one patient diabetes insipidus and panhypopituitarism occurred in association with a tumor of the pineal region in which no tumor was found at autopsy in the pituitary, the hypothalamus, or the supraopticohypophyseal tract. The patient had slight ventral protrusion of the tuberal-infundibular area in association with increased intracranial pressure, and also had infiltration of the pillars of the fornices by the tumor. Possibly, these abnormalities contributed to the development of diabetes insipidus.[40]

Diabetes insipidus is commonly the earliest manifestation of a tumor of the pineal region[36] and is the presenting symptom in virtually all cases of tumor of the chiasmal region.[39] It may precede neurologic or ophthalmologic manifestations of a tumor in either location, by months or even years.[36, 39, 41]

The development of anterior pituitary insufficiency may result in the amelioration of polyuria in a patient with diabetes insipidus of any cause. This is due, at least in part, to glucocorticoid insufficiency. Therefore, a reduction in the severity of diabetes insipidus in a patient with a neoplasm in the pineal or the chiasmal region should suggest the possibility of anterior pituitary insufficiency.

Diabetes insipidus may result in hypernatremia when a patient with this disorder suffers loss of thirst perception, is unable to maintain a sufficiently high water intake in the presence of a very large urine output, or loses consciousness as a result of general anesthesia or an intercurrent illness.[42] Loss of thirst perception may be due to bilateral destruction of hypothalamic thirst centers by a tumor of the chiasmal region or possibly to glucocorticoid deficiency.[42]

Subnormal urinary aldosterone excretion has been reported in 2 patients with lesions localized to the pretectal area by clinical examination and by radiographic contrast studies.[43] Since these patients did not have clinical evidence of aldosterone deficiency, such as hyperkalemia, and since this observation has not been confirmed, the physiologic significance and validity of this finding are open to question.

Anterior Pituitary Insufficiency

Anterior pituitary insufficiency occurs in patients with tumors of the pineal and the chiasmal regions but is even less adequately studied than disorders of sexual maturation and posterior pituitary function, which these people manifest. It is not possible to estimate the frequency with which anterior pituitary dysfunction occurs in these patients. Only a handful of studies contain the kind of clinical and laboratory assessment of endocrine function that is necessary before meaningful conclusions are possible.[36, 40, 41, 44] The few studies that provide such information either deal with few subjects[36, 40, 41, 44] or only with cases in which endocrine dysfunction is present.[36] Reports of large series of patients with tumors of the pineal region, some of which were published before many necessary laboratory tests were available, often assert diagnoses such as hypogonadism, growth retardation, and anterior pituitary insufficiency without presenting either the criteria or the evidence used to establish these findings. Nor is it possible to identify the relative frequency with which deficiencies of the several anterior pituitary hormones occur.

Adrenocorticotropic hormone (ACTH) deficiency and consequent secondary adrenocortical insufficiency may occur in patients with tumors of the pineal region. In one reported case ACTH deficiency appears to have been present in a patient with a mass in the posterior portion of the third ventricle; this 19-year-old man had a low plasma cortisol level at 8 AM, an abnormally small quantity of 17-ketosteroids in the urine, an abnormally small response of urinary 17-hydroxycorticoids to metyrapone, and a normal rise in these urinary steroids to an ACTH infusion.[36] The same authors reported 2 other patients with masses in the pineal region in whom ACTH deficiency is suggested by low plasma cortisol levels in both cases at 8 AM and low urine 17-hydroxycorticoids and 17-ketosteroids in one case. The presence of ACTH deficiency is supported in another case by abnormally low baseline plasma cortisol and urine 17-hydroxycorticosteroid values, which increased in response to an intravenous infusion of ACTH,[40] and suggested in yet another case by low urinary excretion of 17-ketosteroids and 17-ketogenic steroids.[41] The mechanism of ACTH deficiency in patients with tumors of the pineal region has not been studied. It is likely that this abnormality is caused, in at least some patients, by invasion or compression of the hypothalamus or the anterior pituitary, or both.

ACTH deficiency with consequent adrenocortical insufficiency is potentially life threatening, especially in patients who are ill or will be subject to general anesthesia and surgery, as patients with tumors of the pineal region often are. In such cases glucocorticoid therapy may be lifesaving. The symptoms and signs of secondary adrenal insufficiency are nonspecific, and include such common abnormalities as weakness, lethargy, anorexia, nausea, vomiting, fever, and hypotension. The nonspecific nature of these findings may result in failure to make the diagnosis and possibly an underestimate of the frequency of this abnormality in patients under consideration. This may be a serious problem in view of the potential severity of the disorder and the availability of adequate therapy. Clearly, the adrenocortical function of every patient with a tumor of the pineal region must be evaluated. The possibility of secondary adrenocortical insufficiency must be considered when glucocorticoid therapy is discontinued in such patients, since such treatment is frequently required for cerebral edema until adequate decompression of hydrocephalus has been achieved. In such patients secondary adrenocortical insufficiency may be due to both the effects of the tumor and to glucocorticoid therapy.

Similarly it is difficult to determine the frequency with which patients with a tumor of the pineal region experience hypogonadism. As already noted isolated hypogonadism is often asserted to be a feature of tumors of the pineal region. It is not possible to determine whether such delayed sexual maturation in children, or acquired hypogonadism in adults, is due to the putative excess of a pineal antigonadotropic substance or substances, to hypothalamic-pituitary dysfunction, or to the nonspecific effects of systemic disease. The occurrence of hypogonadism in association with deficiencies of other anterior pituitary hormones suggests that the hypogonadism is due to hypothalamic or pituitary dysfunction. One male patient with a tumor of the pineal region, which had invaded the frontal lobes, had clinical and laboratory evidence of diabetes insipidus, hypogonadism (with a low excretion rate of urinary gonadotropins), and secondary adrenocortical insufficiency.[40] Thyroid function tests were abnormally low, but the thyroid gland was atrophic at postmortem examination and primary hypothyroidism was not ruled out. This patient's extensive tumor did not invade the hypothalamus or pituitary gland. (This patient is also discussed above in the section on diabetes insipidus.) Other series, which report hypogonadism in patients with a tumor of the pineal region, do not provide clinical or laboratory evidence to support the diagnosis of hypogonadotropic hypogonadism.

There are no well-documented cases of hypothyroidism in patients with tumors of the pineal region, although hypothyroidism due to hypothalamic-pituitary dysfunction has been said to occur in patients with neoplasms in this area.[22, 45]

There are no studies of growth hormone reserve or prolactin secretion in patients with tumors of the pineal region.

Anterior Pituitary Dysfunction in Patients with Tumors of the Chiasmal Region

Tumors of the chiasmal region have a characteristic presentation, consisting of the triad of diabetes insipidus, visual disturbances, especially bitemporal hemianopsia, and anterior pituitary insufficiency.[39] The endocrine disturbances may be the first manifestations of the tumor, and may antedate visual disturbances and other manifestations of the tumor by months or years.[22, 36, 39] This triad, or the association of diabetes insipidus with either visual disturbances or anterior pituitary insufficiency, should suggest the diagnosis of a tumor of the chiasmal region.

Although anterior pituitary insufficiency is clearly associated with tumors of the chiasmal region, it is difficult to state the frequency of this association or to delineate the relative frequency with which deficiencies of the several anterior pituitary hormones occurs. Hypogonadism, retarded growth, adrenal insufficiency, and hypothyroidism are all alleged to occur in patients with a tumor of the chiasmal region,[36, 39] but careful endocrinologic studies of such patients are available in only 3 patients.[46]

These 3 patients all had diabetes insipidus, manifested by the inability to concentrate urine in response to dehydration, and growth hormone deficiency, with no rise of serum growth hormone levels in response to arginine, insulin, or levodopa. The serum prolactin level was markedly elevated in all 3 patients; 1 of the 2 female patients had galactorrhea. All 3 had low serum levels of luteinizing hormone (LH) and follicle-stimulating hormone (FSH); the single male patient had a low serum testosterone level. Two of the 3 had thyroid stimulating hormone levels that were inappropriately normal, despite low levels of total and free thyroxine. All 3 were thought to have secondary adrenal insufficiency on the basis of low basal plasma or urinary steroids; provocative tests of ACTH reserve were not performed.

Clinical Management

The association of endocrine dysfunction with tumors of both the pineal region and the chiasmal region is important from both a diagnostic and a therapeutic viewpoint.

The development of precocious puberty in a boy should suggest the possibility of a tumor of the pineal region. Such tumors are one of the causes of isolated hypogonadism, diabetes insipidus, and panhypopituitarism in patients in the first three decades of life. Conversely, such patients may develop these endocrine abnormalities while under observation.

The triad of diabetes insipidus, anterior pituitary insufficiency, and visual disturbances (such as bitemporal hemianopsia), or the association of diabetes insipidus with either of the other components of the triad, should suggest the possibility of a tumor of the chiasmal region.

The assessment of endocrine function follows the same principles in patients with the intracranial tumors under discussion as in other patients (Table 8). In all cases, every effort should be made to quantitatively assess the reserve function of the system in question. It is generally unwise to initiate therapy on the basis of suggestive symptoms without careful clinical assessment and laboratory confirmation. The therapy of diabetes insipidus and anterior pituitary insufficiency are generally lifelong undertakings; the diagnosis should be well established before treatment is initiated. In cases where the disorder is life threatening and treatment is urgent, laboratory studies should be obtained before therapy is initiated. For example, in a patient who is thought to have diabetes insipidus, simultaneous serum and urine specimens should be obtained so that sodium concentration and osmolality can be measured at a time when the patient is thought to be dehydrated. Failure to appropriately concentrate urine in response to hypertonicity of serum will confirm the diagnosis of diabetes insipidus. If this abnormality is corrected by the administration of vasopressin, it is intracranial rather than nephrogenic

Table 8. Laboratory Evaluation of Endocrine Function in a Patient with a Tumor of the Pineal or Chiasmal Region

Assessment of Neurohypophyseal Reserve

Determination of osmolality and sodium concentration in serum and urine specimens obtained simultaneously when patient is dehydrated. Failure to appropriately concentrate urine in response to hypertonicity of serum will confirm the diagnosis of diabetes insipidus. Correction of this abnormality by the administration of vasopressin, manifested by the appearance of concentrated urine, will establish that the disorder is intracranial rather than nephrogenic in origin.

Assessment of Adenohypophyseal Reserve

1. Assess *ACTH reserve* and *growth hormone reserve* by measuring plasma cortisol levels and growth hormone levels during an insulin tolerance test. (Alternately ACTH reserve may be assessed by a metyrapone test and growth hormone reserve by the administration of levodopa or arginine.)

2. Assess *gonadotropic function* by a plasma testosterone level in males. If plasma testosterone level is low (or in a female who does not have normal menses) obtain plasma LH and FSH levels.

3. Assess *thyroid function* by measuring the serum thyroxine level. Obtain serum thyroid stimulating hormone (TSH) level if serum thyroxine is low.

4. Assess prolactin secretion by measuring the serum prolactin level.

in origin. Similarly if a patient is thought to have acute adrenocortical insufficiency, plasma cortisol should be determined before a steroid is administered. Under other circumstances, more formal testing will be required. In general this should be performed in consultation with an internist or endocrinologist; successful management of such patients often depends upon collaboration among physicians from several disciplines.

References

1. Wurtman, R. J., Axelrod, J. and Kelly, D. E., *The Pineal.* Academic Press, New York and London (1968).
2. Reiter, R. J. and Fraschini, F., Endocrine aspects of the mammalian pineal gland: a review. *Neuroendocrinology* **5,** 219–255 (1969).
3. Wurtman, R. J., The pineal gland: endocrine interrelationships. *Adv. Intern. Med.* **16,** 155–169 (1970).
4. *The Pineal Gland.* Edited by G. E. W. Wolstenholme and J. Knight. Churchill Livingstone, Edinburgh and London (1971).
5. Reiter, R. J., Comparative physiology: pineal gland. *Annu. Rev. Physiol.* **35,** 305–328 (1973).
6. *Frontiers of Pineal Physiology.* Edited by M. D. Altschule. MIT Press, Cambridge, Mass. and London (1975).
7. Brownstein, M. J., The pineal gland. *Life Sci.* **16,** 1363–1374 (1975).
8. Minneman, K. P. and Wurtman, R. J., Effects of pineal compounds on mammals. *Life Sci.* **17,** 1189–1200 (1975).
9. Reiter, R. J., Endocrine rhythms associated with pineal gland function. *Adv. Exptl. Biol. Med.* **54,** 43–78 (1975).
10. Minneman, K. P. and Wurtman, R. J., The pharmacology of the pineal gland. *Annu. Rev. Pharm. Toxicol.* **16,** 33–51 (1976).
11. Kappers, J. A., The pineal organ: an introduction.[4] pp. 3–34.
12. Axelrod, J., The pineal gland: a neurochemical transducer. *Science* **184,** 1341–1348, (1974).
13. Kitay, J. I. and Altschule, M. D., *The Pineal Gland.* Harvard University Press, Cambridge, Mass. (1954).
14. Fraschini, F., Mess, B. and Martini, L., Pineal gland, melatonin and the control of luteinizing hormone secretion. *Endocrinology* **82,** 919–924 (1968).
15. Pelham, R. W., Vaughan, G. M., Sandock, K. L. and Vaughan, M. K., Twenty-four hour cycle of a melatonin-like substance in the plasma of human males. *J. Clin. Endocrinol. Metab.* **37,** 341–344 (1973).
16. Arendt, J., Paunier, L. and Sizonenko, P. C., Melatonin radioimmunoassay. *J. Clin. Endocrinol. Metab.* **40,** 347–350 (1975).
17. Lynch, H. J., Wurtman, R. J., Moskowitz, M. A., Archer, M. C. and Ho, M. H., Daily rhythm in human urinary melatonin. *Science* **187,** 169–171 (1975).
18. Zacharias, L. and Wurtman, R. J., Blindness: its relation to age of menarche. *Science* **144,** 1154–1155 (1964).
19. David, M., De Ajurriaguerra, J. and Bonis A., Les pubertés précoces des tumeurs cérébrales. *Sem. Hôp. Paris* **67,** 3935–3958 (1957).
20. David, M., Bernard-Weil, E. and Dilenge, D., Les tumeurs de la glande pinéale. *Ann. Endocrinol.* **24,** 287–330 (1963).
21. Jallade, F., Tumeurs de la région pinéale. Problèmes thérapeutiques. Thesis, Lyon (1966).
22. Bovier-Lapierre, M., David, M. and Jeune, M., Manifestations endocriniennes des lésions de la région pinéale chez l'enfant. *Oto.-Neuro.-Ophthalmol.* **45,** 7–16 (1973).
23. Ringertz, N., Nordenstam, H. and Flyger, G., Tumors of the pineal region. *J. Neuropathol. Exp. Neurol.* **13,** 540–561 (1954).
24. Bing, J. F., Globus, J. H., and Simon, H., Pubertas Praecox: a survey of the reported

cases and verified anatomical findings: with particular reference to tumors of the pineal body. *J. Mt. Sinai Hosp.* **4**, 935–965 (1938).

25. Wilkins, L., *Diagnosis and Treatment of Endocrine Disorders in Childhood and Adolescence.* Third edition. CC Thomas, Springfield, Ill, 1965, p. 223.

26. Bierich, J. R., Sexual precocity. *Clin. Endocrinol. Metab.* **4**, 107–142 (1975).

27. Vaitukaitis, J. L., Immunologic and physical characterization of human chorionic gonadotropin (HCG) secreted by tumors. *J. Clin. Endocrinol. Metab.* **37**, 505–514 (1973).

28. Odell, W. D., in discussion of Barnes, N. D., Cloutier, M. D., Hayles, A. B., The central nervous system and precocious puberty, *The Control of the Onset of Puberty.* Edited by Grumbach, M. M., Grave, G. D. and Mayer, F. E., John Wiley, New York, 1974, p. 230.

29. Romshe, C. A. and Sotos, J. F., Intracranial human chorionic gonadotropin-secreting tumor with precocious puberty. *J. Pediatr.* **86**, 250–252 (1975).

30. Case Records of the Massachusetts General Hospital, (Case 38–1975). *N. Engl. J. Med.* **293**, 653–660 (1975).

31. DeGirolami, U. and Schmidek, H., Clinicopathological study of 53 tumors of the pineal region. *J. Neurosurg.* **39**, 455–462 (1973).

32. Braunstein, G. D., Vaitukaitis, J. L., Carbone, P. P. and Ross, G. T., Ectopic production of human chorionic gonadotrophin by neoplasms. *Ann. Intern. Med.* **78**, 39–45 (1973).

33. McArthur, J. W., Toll, G. D., Russfield, A. B., Reiss, A. M., Quinby, W. C. and Baker, W. H., Sexual precocity attributable to ectopic gonadotropin secretion by hepatoblastoma. *Am. J. Med.* **54**, 390–403 (1973).

34. Wurtman, R. J. and Kammer, H., Melatonin synthesis by an ectopic pinealoma. *N. Engl. J. Med.* **274**, 1233–1237 (1966).

35. Wurtman, R. J., Axelrod, J. and Toch, R., Demonstration of hydroxyindole-O-methyl transferase, melatonin, and serotonin in a metastatic parenchymatous pinealoma. *Nature* **204**, 1323–1324 (1964).

36. Puschett, J. B. and Goldberg, M., Endocrinopathy associated with pineal tumor. *Ann. Intern. Med.* **69**, 203–219 (1968).

37. Horrax, G., The role of pinealomas in the causation of diabetes insipidus. *Ann. Surg.* **126**, 725–739 (1947).

38. Stringer, S. W., Diabetes insipidus associated with pinealoma transplant in the tuber cinereum. *Yale J. Biol. Med.* **6**, 375–383 (1934).

39. Rubin, P. and Kramer, S., Ectopic pinealoma: a radiocurable neuroendocrinologic entity. *Radiology* **85**, 512–523 (1965).

40. Booth, C. B., Schwartz, E., Janis, R. and Krueger, E. G., Atypical teratoma (pinealoma): meningoencephalitic and endocrine manifestations. *Neurology* **13**, 999–1010 (1963).

41. Lewis, I., Baxter, D. W. and Stratford, J. G., Atypical teratomas of the pineal. *Can. Med. Assoc. J.* **89**, 103–110 (1963).

42. Ross, E. J. and Christie, S. B. M., Hypernatremia. *Medicine* **48**, 441–473 (1969).

43. Krieger, D. T., Saito, A. and Krieger, H. P., Aldosterone excretion in disease of the pretectum. *Lancet* **2**, 567–570 (1961).

44. Folkes, R. F., The pineal gland and its tumors: with notes on three verified cases. *Bull. LA Neurol. Soc.* **29**, 208–214 (1964).

45. Smith, R. A., Pineal tumors. *Univ. Mich. Med. Bull.* **27**, 33–43 (1961).

46. Spiegel, A. M., DiChiro, G., Gorden, P., Ommaya, A. K., Kolins, J. and Pomeroy, T. C., Diagnosis of radiosensitive hypothalamic tumors without craniotomy: endocrine and neuroradiologic studies of intracranial atypical teratomas. *Ann. Intern. Med.* **85**, 290–293 (1976).

47. Russell, W. O. and Sachs, E., Pinealoma: a clinicopathologic study of seven cases with a review of the literature. *Arch. Pathol.* **35**, 869–888 (1943).

48. Dayan, A. D., Marshall, A. H. E., Miller, A. A., Pick, F. J. and Rankin, N. E., Atypical teratomas of the pineal and hypothalamus. *J. Pathol. Bacteriol.* **92**, 1–28 (1966).

CHAPTER FOUR
Neuroradiology of the Pineal Region

Charles B. Grossman
Carlos F. Gonzalez   Hershey and Philadelphia, PA

FUNDAMENTAL ANATOMIC CONSIDERATIONS are necessary for the interpretation of radiologic studies directed to the pineal region. The pineal gland projects into the quadrigeminal plate cistern. It is superior to the corpora quadrigemina and just anterior to and beneath the splenium of the corpus callosum (Fig. 24).

Normal Peneal Region Radiology

Conventional skull radiography demonstrates pineal gland calcification in approximately 60% of the population of the United States over 20 years of age. Calcification related to the habenular commissure is seen in approximately half of these patients (Fig. 25). Pineal calcification is rarely seen before 6 years of age. The upper limit of normal for the diameter of the roentgenologically normal pineal gland is 10 mm.[1] The normal pineal gland should be midline on frontal projection and fall within measurable normal parameters on lateral projection.[1,2]

The extraordinary ability of computed tomography (CT scanning) to directly visualize brain structures with a high degree of accuracy and without significant risk establishes this procedure as the single most important radiographic study in the investigation of abnormalities of the pineal region. The sharp detail of the pineal gland on CT scanning is due to the contrasting densities of the often calcified pineal gland, projecting into the cerebrospinal fluid of the quadrigeminal plate cistern and its proximity to the cerebrospinal fluid of the third ventricle (Fig. 26). The pineal gland rarely measures greater than 100 mm^2 on CT scans.[3,4]

The close relationship of the pineal gland to the third ventricle gives

Assistant Professor of Radiology, Milton S. Hershey Medical Center, and Associate Professor of Medicine, Hahnemann Medical College

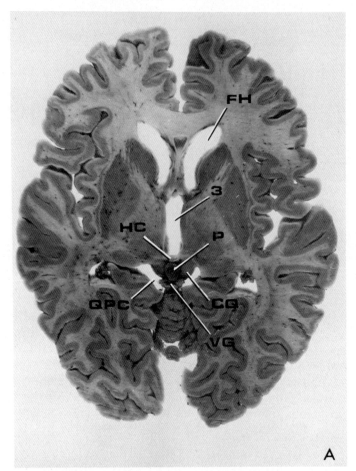

A

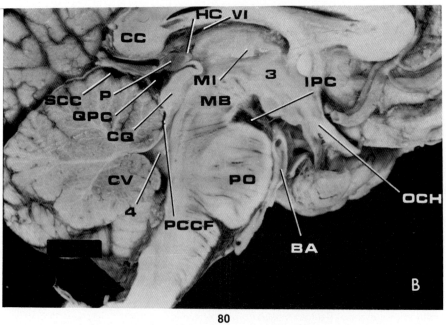

B

80

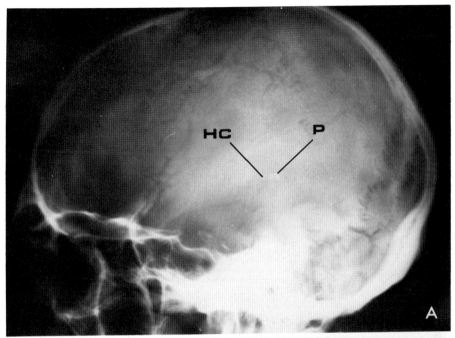

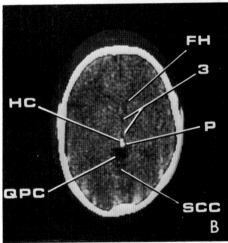

Figure 25. **A.** Conventional skull x-ray, lateral projection, showing habenular calcification (HC) and calcified pineal gland (P). Note the normal sella turcica. **B.** Computed tomogram, same case as A. In addition to the habenular (HC) and pineal (P) calcifications, brain anatomy is now clearly visualized. The massa intermedia is seen dividing the third ventricle (3). The pineal gland projects into the quadrigeminal plate cistern (QPC). SCC = superior cerebellar cistern, FH = frontal horn, lateral ventricle.

Figure 24. **A.** Horizontal section of brain approximating the CT section through the pineal gland. **B.** Midsagittal section shows the pineal gland (P) within the quadrigeminal plate cistern (QPC), the third ventricle (3), the corpora quadrigemina (CQ) inferior to the pineal gland, the vein of Galen (VG), and the frontal horn of the lateral ventricle (FH). On sagittal section, the superior-posterior relationship of the splenium (CC) of the corpus callosum is well demonstrated. PCCF = precentral cerebellar fissure, SCC = superior cerebellar cistern, IPC = interpeduncular cistern, BA = basilar artery anterior to the pons, O-CH = optic chiasm, VI = velum interpositum, CV = cerebellar vermis, 4 = fourth ventricle, MB = midbrain, MI = massa intermedia.

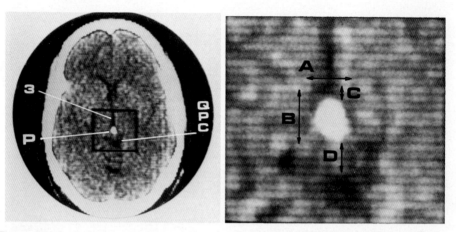

Figure 26.   Left. Normal pineal level CT scan. **Right.** Magnification of enclosed area. 3 = third ventricle, QPC = quadrigeminal plate cistern, P = pineal gland. The pineal gland area approximation is the product of the coronal (A) and sagittal (B) diameters corrected for magnification. The average normal pineal gland area is 34 mm². The distance of the anterior margin of the pineal gland to the posterior margin of the third ventricle (C) is usually less than 6 mm in the normal patient. The distance between the posterior margin of the pineal gland and the quadrigeminal plate cistern (D) is usually less than 8 mm in the normal adult.[3]

added emphasis to the value of ventriculography and pneumoencephalography in this area (Fig. 27).

Arteriography demonstrates arteries and veins related to the quadrigeminal plate cistern, splenium of the corpus callosum, and cerebellar vermis (Fig. 28). In addition the type of regional vascularity can be studied.[5]

Radionuclide scanning plays a significant role in investigations of pineal region abnormality. Both flow and static scan techniques are helpful in evaluating the pineal region.

Abnormal Pineal Region Radiology

Conventional skull radiography of patients with pineal tumors may demonstrate premature calcification, irregular or amorphous-type calcifications, or an abnormally large pineal gland (Fig. 29). In addition the pineal calcification may be low in position due to hydrocephalus. Erosion of the dorsum sellae or widening of the sutures of the cranial vault represents evidence for raised intracranial pressure (Fig. 30).

Computed tomographic scans of pineal masses will often demonstrate a mass greater than 100 mm² in area, producing distortion of or possibly obstruction of the third ventricle, with resultant hydrocephalus[6] (Figs. 30 and 31). The density of the mass may vary and contrast enhancement may possibly be required, i.e., the intravenous injection of a water-soluble iodinated contrast medium, for visualization (Fig. 31). Intraventricular spread or seeding may be demonstrated by the intravenous injection of contrast medium (Fig. 31B).

It is often necessary to enhance the CT scan by injecting a contrast medium because augmentation of densities may be required to demonstrate

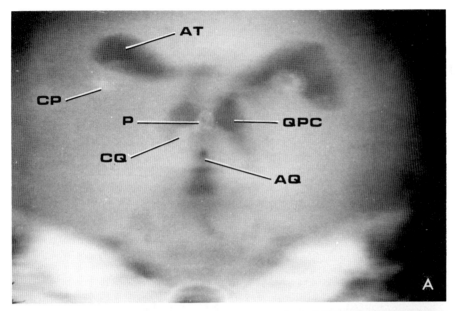

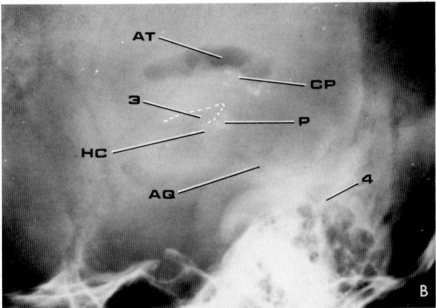

Figure 27. Normal pneumoencephalogram, frontal and lateral projections. **A.** Frontal pneu-
motomogram, sitting position, ventricular and cisternal air. Pineal gland (p) in quadrigeminal
plate cistern (QPC), superior colliculus (CQ). **B.** Lateral conventional projection, sitting
position, ventricular air only. Third ventricle suprapineal recess (3) is superior to pineal gland
(P). Habenular calcification (HC) interposed between the pineal gland and third ventricle. AT
= atrium lateral ventricle, CP = calcified choroid plexus, 4 = fourth ventricle, AQ =
aqueduct.

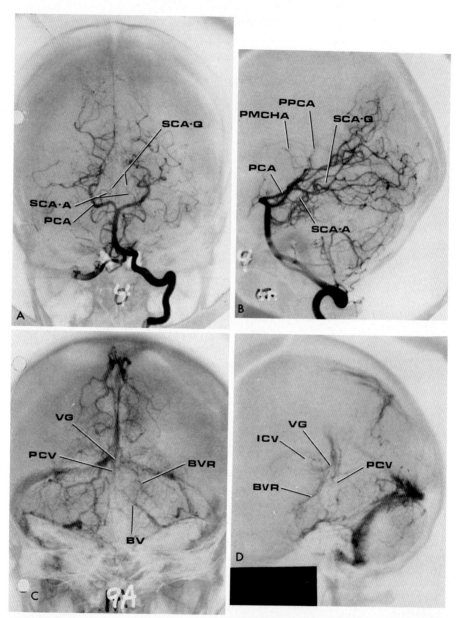

Figure 28. Normal pineal region vascular anatomy. Arterial and venous phases vertebral angiogram. **A.** Frontal and **B.** lateral projections, arterial phase. Superior cerebellar artery, ambient (SCA-A) and quadrigeminal (SCA-Q) segments. These segments correspond to the appropriate cisterns within which the superior cerebellar and posterior cerebral arteries course around the brainstem. Posterior medial choroidal artery (PMCHA) and posterior pericallosal artery (PPCA) seen on lateral projection only. The PMCHA and PPCA are proximal branches of the posterior cerebral artery (PCA). **C.** Frontal and **D.** lateral projections, venous phase. Precentral cerebellar vein (PCV) in the precentral cerebellar fissure. VG = vein of Galen, BV = brachial vein in the precentral cerebellar fissure, seen on frontal projection only. BVR = basal vein of Rosenthal, ICV = internal cerebral vein. The ICV courses in the velum interpositum (roof of the third ventricle). Note the vein of Galen superimposed over the torcula herophili in the frontal projection. The infratentorial analog of the basal vein of Rosenthal is more accurately named the posterior mesencephalic vein.[1]

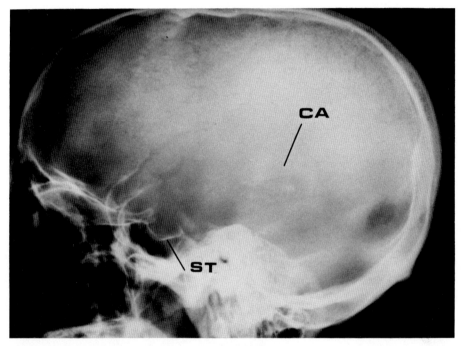

Figure 29. Conventional skull x-ray showing pinealoma in a 21-year-old male. Admission skull x-ray. Lateral projection, shows subsequently proved pinealoma, large zone of irregular calcification (CA) in pineal region, and eroded sella turcica (ST).

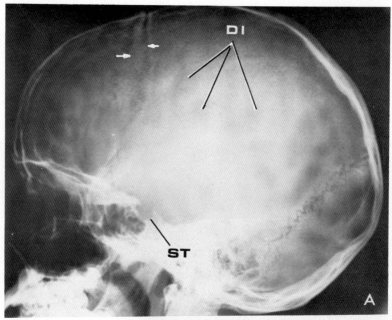

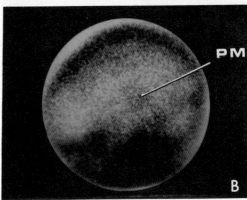

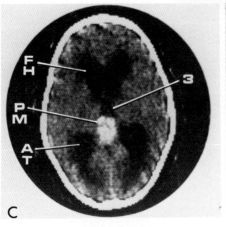

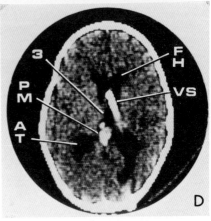

Figure 30.   A. Conventional skull x-ray, lateral projection, showing widened coronal suture (arrows) in a 7-year-old female admitted for nausea, vomiting, and Parinaud's syndrome. Lamina dura of sella turcica (ST) is eroded, and there are prominent digital impressions (DI). **B.** Radionuclide scan, left lateral view, showing large area of abnormal activity in pineal region (PM). **C.** CT scan pineal level, no contrast injection, admission study, shows 400 mm² dense pineal region mass (PM) obstructing and distorting the third ventricle (3). Hydrocephalic frontal horns (FH) and atria (AT) of the lateral ventricles. **D.** Postirradiation therapy, 5,200 rads in divided doses, and ventricular shunt (VS). The mass diameter is now approximately half that pretreatment. Reduction of hydrocephalus. The complementary role of conventional x-ray films of the skull (raised intracranial pressure), radionuclide scan (abnormal vascularity or blood-brain barrier breakdown), and CT scan (calcified obstructing pineal region mass) for diagnosis and evaluation of therapeutic results is clearly demonstrated. (Courtesy of John Gareiss, M.D., Lancaster General Hospital, Lancaster, Pennsylvania.)

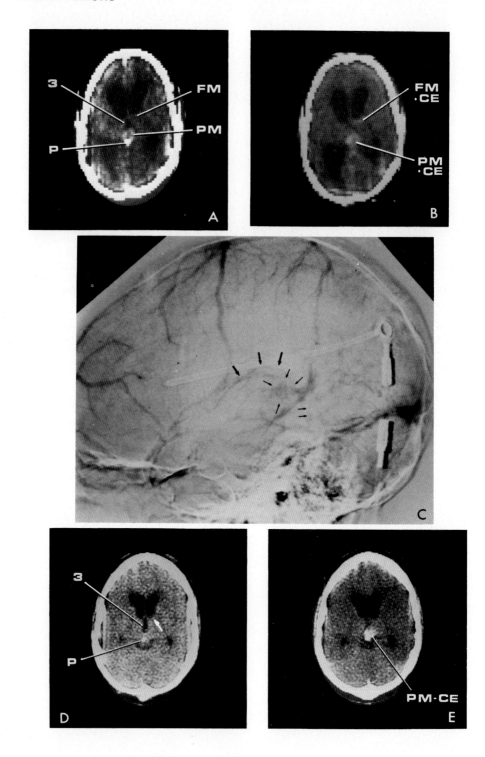

Figure 31. Pineoblastoma in a 21-year-old male presenting with headache, nausea and vomiting, and Parinaud's syndrome. CT scans pre- and post-treatment, and preirradiation angiogram. **A.** CT scan, preinjection, showing calcified pineal mass (PM) and more densely calcified pineal gland (P), obstructed distorted third ventricle (3), mass effect on right frontal horn (FM), and a marked degree of hydrocephalus. The posterior aspect of the third ventricle is separated 14 mm from the anterior margin of the pineal gland. **B.** CT scan, same level, intravenous contrast enhancement, same day. Tumor density has increased (PM-CE). Intraventricular tumor deposit contrast enhancement (FM-CE). **C.** Right brachial arteriogram, early venous phase, lateral projection, postventricular shunt. Tumor neovascularity (four medium size arrows). Posteriorly displaced precentral cerebellar vein (paired small arrows) and elevated internal cerebral vein (three large arrows). The arteriogram has confirmed the presence of a neoplasm. **D.** Postirradiation CT scan (4,000 rads). The ventricular shunt has been removed. Decreased third ventricular distortion (3) and decreased tumor density are noted. The anterior margin of the pineal gland (P) measures 7 mm from the posterior margin of the third ventricle. Right frontal horn mass effect is no longer present (arrow). The degree of hydrocephalus had moderately decreased. **E.** Postirradiation CT scan with intravenous contrast enhancement (PM-CE). The size of the tumor is essentially the same as on scan B, however, tumor density has decreased and the mass is more eccentric at this time. The right frontal horn tumor deposit is no longer present.

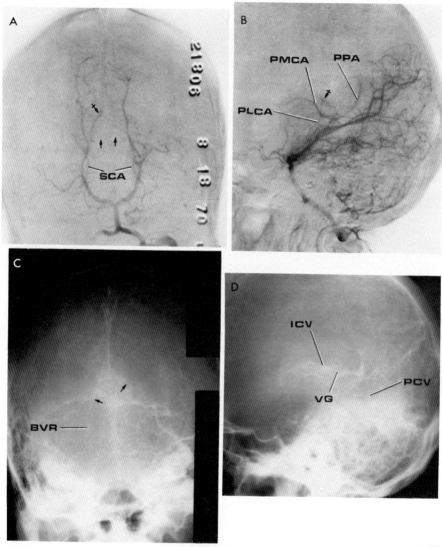

Figure 32. Pinealoma. Patient is a 20-year-old male, now presenting with paraparesis, who had a known posterior third ventricular tumor at the age of 18, which was radiated at that time. **A–D.** Vertebral arteriography, first admission study, arterial and venous phase. **A–B.** Arterial phase, frontal (A) and lateral (B) projections show laterally displaced superior cerebellar artery segments related to quadrigeminal plate cistern (SCA). Enlarged encased posterior medial choroidal artery (PMCA) supplying tumor neovascularity (crossed arrow). Widened sweep posterior pericallosal artery (PPA) indicates hydrocephalus. PLCA = posterior lateral choroidal artery. **C–D.** Venous phase, frontal (C) and lateral (D) projections show laterally displaced basal vein of Rosenthal (BVR) segments related to the quadrigeminal plate cistern (arrows), elevated distal internal cerebral vein (ICV) and vein of Galen (VG). Dorsally displaced precentral cerebellar vein (PCV). **E.** Pneumoencephalogram, sitting position,

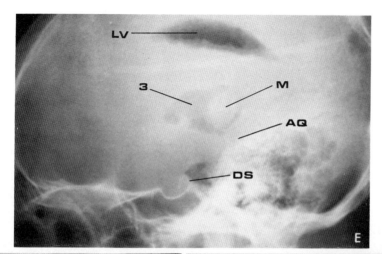

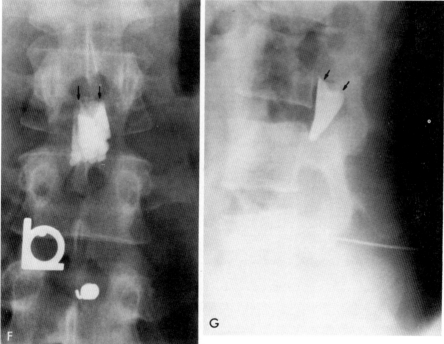

lateral projection, first admission study, Mass (M) distorts and displaces the posterior third ventricle (3) forward and upward. Aqueduct of Sylvius (AQ), hydrocephalic lateral ventricles and eroded lamina dura of dorsum sella (DS). Arterial and venous correlates of a pineal region mass producing obstructive hydrocephalus are compared to the pneumoencephalographic result. Mass expansion of the quadrigeminal plate cistern (PCA) (SCA) (BVR), distortion of the posterior third ventricle (PMCA) (ICV), dorsal displacement of the precentral cerebellar fissure (PCV), and hydrocephalus (PPA) correlate well with the pneumoencephalographic result. **F–G.** Myelogram, Trendelenberg position, frontal and lateral projections, second admission. Intradural extramedullary mass (arrows) obstructing the subarachnoid space. Pathologic tissue, pinealoma.

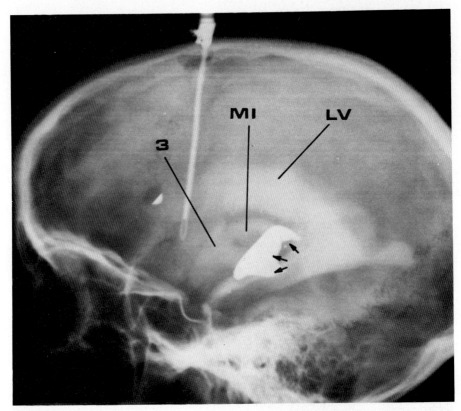

Figure 33 Combined Conray-Pantopaque ventriculography shows pinealoma (arrows) obstructing and distorting the third ventricle (3). MI = massa intermedia, LV = hydrocephalic lateral ventricle.

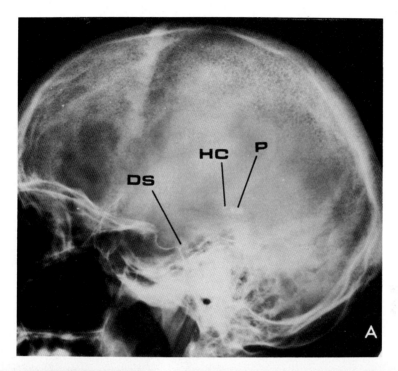

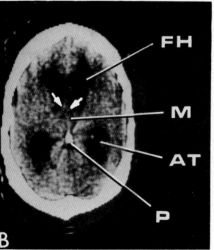

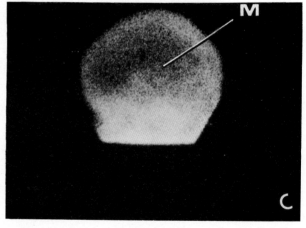

Figure 34. Ectopic pinealoma in a 34-year-old male with a 1-year history of headaches and impotence, bitemporal hemianopsia, and an allergy to x-ray contrast material. **A.** Lateral skull x-ray shows eroded dorsum clinoid (DS), lamina dura of the sella turcica, and slightly low-positioned calcified pineal gland (P) and habenular commissure (HC). **B.** Pineal level CT scan shows calcified pineal gland (P), mass (M) obliterating the third ventricle, mass extending into the region of the foramen of Monro (arrows), hydrocephalic frontal horn (FH), and atrium (AT) of the lateral ventricle. Injection-enhanced scan could not be done because of the patient's allergy. **C.** ⁹⁹ᵐTc radionuclide brain scan, left lateral projection shows increased activity in the suprasellar location extending posteriorly to the pineal location (M). **D.** Hanging head air ventriculogram, lateral midline tomogram showing eroded dorsum sella

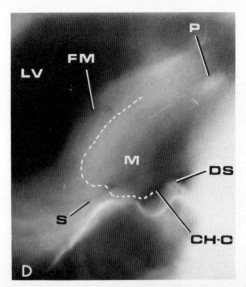

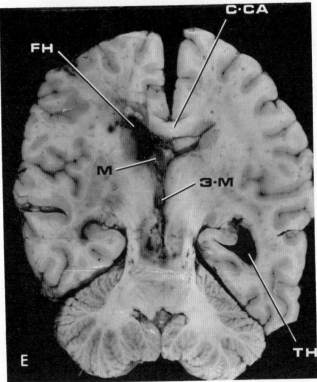

(DS), mass (dotted line) distorting chiasmatic cistern (CH-C), and an interhemispheric sulcus (S), and invading the foramen of Monro (FM). LV = hydrocephalic lateral ventricle. **E.** Brain section roughly corresponding to the pineal level CT scan. The tumor had been biopsied and the ventricles were shunted. A mass (M) obstructs the foramen of Monro and is invading the third ventricle (3-M). Hemorrhage in the left frontal horn (FH) and right temporal horn (TH) of the lateral ventricles, possibly secondary to operative intervention. C-CA = corpus callosum. The eroded lamina dura indicates raised intracranial pressure. The low pineal gland position is consistent with hydrocephalus. CT scan indicates a mass obstructing the foramen of Monro and radionuclide scan indicates a blood-brain barrier breakdown or abnormal vascularity. Ventriculogram demonstrates the extent of the mass to sagittal dimension. The complementary roles of the various procedures are well demonstrated here, particularly with reference to x-ray contrast allergy.

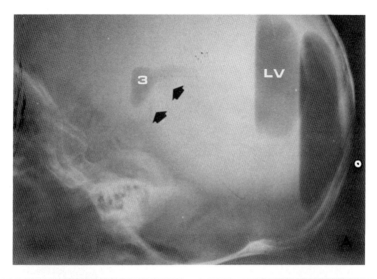

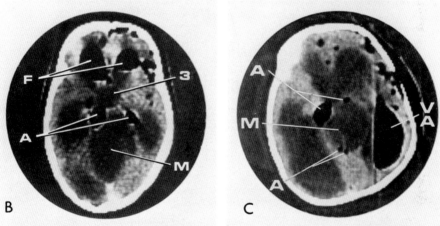

Figure 35. Quadrigeminal plate cistern subarachnoid cyst in a 7-month-old female, with an enlarging head but neurologically normal. **A.** Conventional air ventriculogram, lateral projection, brow down, shows mass (arrows) distorting the third ventricle (3). LV = hydrocephalic lateral ventricles. **B.** CT scan, brow up, showing 38-mm diameter water-density mass (M) obstructing third ventricle (3). Air can be seen in both frontal horns (F); subarachnoid air (A) surrounds mass. **C.** CT scan, left side down, shows patent foramen of Monro, air-filled enlarged atrium of right lateral ventricle (VA), and subarachnoid air (A) surrounding the mass (M). The presumed cyst does not communicate with the ventricular or cisternal fluid compartments. In addition to demonstrating ventricular and cisternal abnormality, the CT pneumatogram demonstrates details of nonair-filled structures with respect to size, shape, position, and density.

detail. For instance, a tissue density mass may extend into the area of the velum interpositum or directly lateral to it, without displacing the ventricular system, as seen in horizontal sections (Figs. 31D and E). Injection enhancement of a vascular mass extending into these locations would localize the spread of the mass.

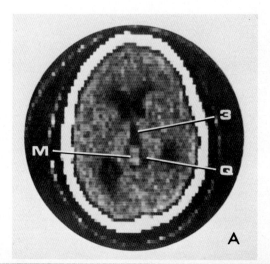

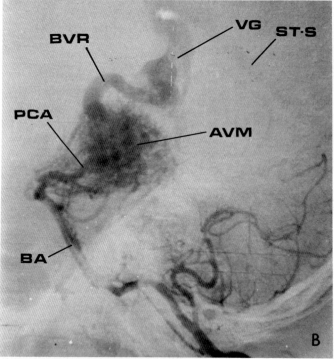

Figure 36. A. CT scan, pineal level in an 11-year-old male with a long history of cranial nerve signs, nausea, vomiting, and papilledema. M = rectangular tissue-density mass within the quadrigeminal plate cistern (Q), 3 = dilated third ventricle. **B.** Left vertebral arteriogram, lateral projection, from same patient, shows large interpeduncular AV malformation (AVM) draining to the vein of Galen (VG). The vein of Galen is responsible for the rectangular mass in (A). ST-S = stright sinus, BVR = basal vein of Rosenthal, PCA = posterior cerebral artery.

Progress in the tumor's course can be well demonstrated by CT scanning, particularly with injection enhancement. Regression in the size of the pineal tumor of unknown tissue type is well demonstrated by Figure 30D. Figure

31E shows eccentric regrowth of a pineoblastoma following irradiation.

Ventriculography is usually the method of choice for opacification of ventricular pathways in these particular patients because of the usual clinical presentation of ventricular obstruction. Ventriculography using either negative or positive contrast material will clearly demonstrate the exact relationship of the mass to the posterior third ventricle (Figs. 32E and 33). Ectopic pinealoma is an unusual presentation, often found related to the anterior third ventricle (Fig. 34). Brow-up ventriculography is helpful in the latter situation. Growth of the tumor in directions somewhat remote from the ventricular system or quadrigeminal plate cistern would obviously not be sharply demonstrated by ventriculography alone. Combined ventriculography and CT scanning can be extremely valuable[6] (Fig. 35).

Vertebral angiography is quite helpful in demonstrating the nature or lack of vascularity of a particular mass in the posterior third ventricular location. Of particular interest is the exclusion of an AV malformation (Fig. 36) or of a vein of Galen aneurysm. Vascular displacement helps to localize lesions. Separation of the arteries in the distal ambient and quadrigeminal plate cisterns and abnormal configuration of the posterior medial choroidal artery (Figs. 32A and B) and tumor vascularity (Figs. 31C and 32B) are demonstrated. Extension of the mass into the third ventricle location anteriorly would tend to elevate the internal cerebral vein and inferior extension would tend to posteriorly displace the precentral cerebellar vein[1, 5] (Figs. 31C and 32D).

Radionuclide scanning may demonstrate an abnormal zone of activity in the pineal or posterior third ventricular location (Fig. 30B). Radionuclide scanning is helpful as a screening procedure and may be quite helpful if a patient is allergic to intravenous contrast material (Fig. 34C), or in a patient with a highly calcified pineal tumor in which injection may fail to demonstrate enhanced contrast (Fig. 30B).

Finally, a discourse on radiology of pineal tumors would be incomplete without demonstration, myelographically, of tumor deposition in the spinal subarachnoid space (Figs. 32F and G). The intracranial analogous situation of subarachnoid tumor deposition has already been demonstrated (Fig. 31B).

Summary

Various procedures for the neuroradiologic diagnosis of pineal tumors have been discussed. The screening procedure of choice is the CT scan; however, the complementary roles of other methods are discussed, with particular emphasis on normal anatomy. Decisions regarding choice and order of procedure depend on a variety of factors. Conventional skull x-ray studies, conventional CT scan, and radionuclide imaging are noninvasive techniques. Risks of contrast allergy and risks of arterial and subarachnoid or ventricular invasive procedures must be weighed against the potential diagnostic yield. Considerations, such as operability or postirradiation status, will influence the choice of diagnostic procedures.

References

1. *Radiology of the Skull and Brain.* Edited by T. H. Newton and D. G. Potts. C. V. Mosby, St Louis (1971).
2. Taveras, J. M., and Wood, E. H., *Diagnostic Neuroradiology.* Williams and Wilkins, Baltimore, (1964).
3. Grossman, C. G., Gonzalez, C. F. and Lee, F. K., Normal anatomy and pathological conditions of the pineal region — a comparative study utilizing CT scanning and conventional neuroradiological methods. *Neuroradiology* **9,** 284 (1975).
4. Gonzalez, C. F., Grossman, C. B., and Palacios, E., *Brain and Orbital Computed Tomography.* John Wiley, New York (1976).
5. Sones, P. J., and Hoffman, J. C., Angiography of tumors involving the posterior third ventricle. *Am. J. Roentgenol.* **124,** 241–250 (1975).
6. Greitz, T. and Hindmarsh, T., Computer assisted tomography of intracranial CSF circulation using a water-soluble contrast medium. *Acta Radiol. Diag.* **15,** 497–507 (1974).

CHAPTER FIVE
Surgical Management of Pineal Region Tumors

Henry H. Schmidek   Philadelphia, Pennsylvania

NEOPLASMS IN THE REGION of the pineal gland cause symptoms when they invade or compress adjacent structures, producing local effects or tumor cells spread to distant sites (Fig. 37). If the cerebral aqueduct becomes involved, intracranial hypertension develops. If the superior colliculus and pretectal region become involved, characteristic eye signs occur and when the cerebellum is involved, dysmetria, hypotonia, and intention tremor are manifest. Ectopic tumors extend from the pineal region to involve the anterior third ventricle and parasellar structures, resulting in optic atrophy, bitemporal hemianopsia, diabetes insipidus, and panhypopituitarism. Altered consciousness may be present, due either to intracranial hypertension or to hypothalamic invasion by the tumor. Intradural metastases to the spinal cord or cauda equina, or hematogenous metastases to structures outside the nervous system, are other manifestations of pineal region tumors.

Although there are several diagnostic possibilities that may explain a lesion in the posterior third ventricle, the crucial differential is that which must be made between benign and malignant lesions. Approximately 10% of the lesions in this area are truly benign. These are the pineocytomas, cysts, vein of Galen malformations, and tentorial meningiomas. Another 5% to 10% are relatively benign and include dermoid tumors and low-grade gliomas. The remaining 80% to 85% are highly malignant neoplasms. With increasing neuroradiologic sophistication, at least some of these benign tumors should be identifiable preoperatively with a high degree of certainty and have been shown to represent a particularly favorable subgroup for direct surgical intervention.

Skull radiographs in 50% of pineal tumors show changes caused by chronic intracranial hypertension. In addition abnormalities in the amount

Professor and Chairman, Department of Neurosurgery, Hahnemann Medical College and Hospital, Philadelphia, Pennsylvania

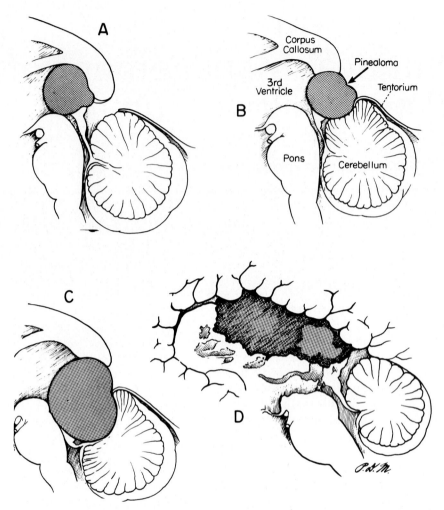

Figure 37   Schematic representation of the types of pineal region tumors and their local extension. (Reproduced by permission from Poppen, J. L., The right occipital approach to a pinealoma. *J. Neurosurg.* **25,** 706–710 (1966).)

and configuration of calcification in the pineal region may indicate the presence of an aneurysm, dermoid, meningioma, or low-grade glioma. Chest radiography excludes a malignancy of lung or one that may have metastasized to lung and brain. Computerized tomography (CT) indicates the size and position of the lesion, the presence of a calcific, cystic, or hemorrhagic component in the neoplasm; and the degree of associated hydrocephalus. The CT scan also provides evidence of tumor extension into the lateral ventricles or parasellar structures. Further investigation includes angiographic study of both the carotid and vertebral systems to characterize the nature and vascularity of the posterior ventricular lesion, and the relationship of the deep venous structures to the tumor. It should be possible to exclude or identify benign lesions, such as aneurysms of the vein of Galen, meningiomas arising from the superior tela choroidea (velum interpositum), or at the junction of the free edge of the tentorium and the inferior margin of the falx. Some radiologic features make it possible to diagnose the site and nature of these tumors (see Chapter 4).

Cytologic examination of spinal fluid obtained at pneumoencephalography, ventriculography, or shunting is crucial, since malignant cells in spinal fluid will establish the nature of the posterior ventricular lesion. The propensity of pineal tumors to seed cerebrospinal fluid pathways appears to be particularly characteristic of germinomas and results in symptomatic spinal metastases in 8% of pineal tumors. For this reason, there may be a place for the myelographic investigation of the spinal subarachnoid space, even in the asymptomatic patient with a posterior third ventricular tumor.

Surgical Alternatives

Since pineal tumors are perhaps the most dangerous intracranial mass to excise surgically, there has been an ongoing debate for the last half century concerning their management.[1] This debate centers on whether it is in the patient's best interest to explore these lesions at the time they are diagnosed and to attempt to remove those that are benign or whether to treat the obstructive hydrocephalus with a shunt and irradiate the tumor without histologic characterization. The high morbidity and mortality associated with their surgical exploration is cited as ample reason to choose the latter approach in the management of pineal tumors.

Surgical Procedures Other Than Tumor Biopsy or Removal

Since they are a particularly difficult problem, pineal tumors have been a technical challenge to several generations of neurosurgeons. Few therapeutic options were available to the surgeon before 1940. The predominant symptom, obstructive hydrocephalus, was usually managed by subtemporal decompression as an alternative to direct tumor excision. Ward[2] collected 14 cases treated by subtemporal decompression and irradiation. Two of these patients failed to respond to treatment and proved to have cysts obstructing the aqueduct, 6 had malignant gliomas, and 6 were alive and well 6 to 16 years after surgery. These results represented a significant improvement over those reported when these tumors were removed surgically. Third ventriculostomy produced by a puncture of the lamina terminalis of the third ventricle was used, after 1936, to relieve obstructive hydrocephalus. The aperture created in the anterior third ventricle often closed within a short time, and for this reason this operation was used infrequently after the Torkildsen procedure of ventriculocisternostomy was introduced.

Torkildsen, in 1948,[3] reported his experience with 8 patients in whom pineal tumors were treated by diverting the obstructed spinal fluid from the lateral ventricle to the cisterna magna with a catheter. Three were alive and well $7^{1}/_{2}$, $4^{1}/_{2}$, and 2 years, respectively, after operation. Only 1 patient with a medulloblastoma in the pineal region and in extremis at the time of surgery, died postoperatively.

In the last three decades there have been several technical improvements in the shunt procedures and mechanical systems used for diverting spinal fluid. At the present time ventriculoatrial or ventriculoperitoneal shunts are used most often. These shunts have interposed valves that permit intraventricular pressure to be reduced to a predetermined extent. They may also include filters to reduce chances of seeding malignant cells from an intracranial tumor into the bloodstream or peritoneal cavity. These operations can be performed with a mortality rate less than 5% in patients with pineal tumors and, when combined with irradiation, many long-term survivals have resulted. Although the pineal mass is not verified histologically, the success of this tactic establishes a standard of comparison for other available surgical options.

Biopsy or Excision of Pineal Tumors

Infratentorial Approach

Since the early decades of this century, a variety of operations has been devised to remove tumors situated in the posterior third ventricle. In 1971 Stein[4] reintroduced the posterior fossa supracerebellar approach to the pineal region. This approach was tried and discussed by Horsley[5] in 1910. His results in 2 cases explored through the posterior fossa convinced him that given the opportunity he would use another approach, preferably supratentorial, in future explorations. In 1926 Krause[6] formally described the infratentorial supracerebellar approach to the pineal region. This operation had the advantage of (a) excluding a cerebellar tumor misdiagnosed as a pineal mass, a not uncommon occurrence at that time, and (b) avoiding the deep venous system usually situated dorsal and lateral to these tumors. Injury to the deep veins is the main cause of surgical morbidity associated with operations in this region (Table 9).

The vein of Galen drains the medial areas of the diencephalon, the basal ganglia, the midbrain, the medial aspect of the hemisphere, and the corpus callosum, and if injured, results in fatal venous infarction within this drainage area. Division of the internal occipital vein often results in a permanent homonymous hemianopsia.[13]

Stein[4] reported his experience with 8 patients using the supracerebellar approach. The essentials of the procedure are that it is performed in the sitting position, preoperative ventricular drainage is used, a suboccipital craniectomy, extending to the transverse sinus and torcula, is performed, and the arch of C1 is removed. The tentorium is retracted upwards and the bridging veins from the upper surfaces of the cerebellum can be sacrificed without reported sequelae. Under magnification, the arachnoid of the quadrigeminal region is opened, exposing the tumor and deep veins above and lateral to it. The tumor is first aspirated and then, if the lesion is not cystic, the capsule is opened and the tumor decompressed. Only in an encapsulated lesion that dissects easily from surrounding structures is resection attempted. Should the cerebrospinal fluid obstruction not have been relieved at this point, either a ventriculocisternostomy or another type of shunt can be

Table 9.   Results – Surgical Management Pineal Region Tumors (1910-1976)

	No. of Cases	Approach	Findings	Operative Results
Horsley[5] (1910)	2	Infratentorial	—	Postoperative death
Roschach[7] (1913)	1	Infratentorial	—	Postoperative death
Brunner[8] (1913)	1	Supratentorial, section of corpus callosum	Suspected tumor	—
Pussepp[9] (1914)	1	Supratentorial	Cyst	—
Pecker[10]	1	—	1	Alive 7 years postop
VanWagenen[11] (1931)	1	Transventricular	3×3.5cm glioma	Subtotal radical removal Postop hemiplegia, coma – improved. Alive and well 1$^1/_2$ yr later
Sachs[12] (1931)	1	—	Cystic tumor	—
Harris[13] (1932)	1	Dandy	Pinealoma	Radical removal. Recurred 9 mo
Dandy[14] (1933)	10	Dandy	—	7 consecutive deaths, 8th patient dead in 3 mo. Two survivals at 4 mo, 30 mo.
Horrax[15] (1937)	1	Supratentorial and occipital lobectomy	Large tumor	—
Pratt[16] (1938)	1	—	Teratoma	Alive 3$^1/_2$ yrs postop
Baggenstoss[17] (1939)	1	Two-stage operation – transcallosal and subtentorial	—	—
Russel[18] (1944)			—	29 deaths (Review of 58 cases – 32 operated)
Torkildsen[3] (1948)	8	Ventriculocisternostomy	—	1 death
Olivecrona[19] (1967)	41	—	—	20 deaths
Horrax[20] (1950)	11	—	—	8 deaths; 3 alive and well
Rand[21] (1953)	17	Dandy 16; Van-Wagenen 1	—	MR 70%
Cummins[21] (1956)	32	—		MR 34%; shunt MR 5%
Kunicki[23] (1959)	8	Dandy and hypothermia	Morbidity – av. hospitalization 4 mo. Marked degrees of deficit	MR 25%, 2 postop deaths; 2 deaths within 2 yr; 4 functional survivors
Suzuki[24] (1965)	17	14 transcallosal Morbidity 60% operative MR 10% 3 transventricular and hypothermia and ventricular drainage preop +	10% benign and low grade Postop ± postop shunt and rads	35% deaths in 1 yr (now favors shunt and rads)
Poppen[25] (1968)	13 of biopsy or subtotal removal of 45 cases listed	Occipital and transtentorial approach	Operated 8; 5 died within 1 yr	Vegetative state postop
Stein[4] (1971) (1975 – 14 cases total benign 20% 1 postop death	6	Postorior fossa, supracerebellar approach preop ventriculostomy, no operative MR	With additional cases has benign lesions in less than 20% of cases.	6 cases – 2 subtotal radical removal. Postop aseptic meningitis, cerebellar ataxia

Table 9—*Continued*

	No. of Cases	Approach	Findings	Operative Results
			Case 1 Teratoma	
			Case 2 epidermoid	
			Case 3 shunt and rads—op with progression; astrocytoma	
			Case 4 cyst in quadrigeminal region	
			Case 5 shunt and rads–subtotal removal—shunt	
			Case 6 atypical teratoma—shunt from III–IV and rads.	
Jamieson[21] (1971)	8	Poppen approach and section of tentorium Case 1, injury to occipital lobe, resected	Case 1 pineocytoma first Rx for shunt and XRT, op with recurrence Case 2 cyst—immediate op—good result Case 3 atypical teratoma—no rads Case 4 atypical teratoma—± XRT postop Case 5 atypical teratoma— Case 6 Case 7 thrombosed vein of Galen aneurysm—no details Case 8 atypical teratoma—no details	
Kirsch[27] (1970)	1	2 courses XRT and shunts	Epidermoid	Recurred postop shunt
MGH series[28] (1973)	Dandy			
Conway[29] (1973)	6	Stereotactic biopsy; 2 cases with cryo lesion		No reported morbidity or mortality
Sugita[30] (1975)	10	Stereotactic biopsy Ventriculography Use of evoked EEG to detect tumor margeins	Pinealoma 4 Gua 3 Terato CA 1 Medullo 1	No reported morbidity or mortality
Lazar[31] (1974)	6	Poppen approach with tentorial section	15% (1 cast—met CA), 1 death in 5 mo	Selected cases meningioma-dx preop multiple shunts and rads, surgery vein of Galen lesion shunt and rads astrocytoma, postop rads

performed. Alternatively the patient is kept on ventricular drainage for several days and a shunt performed as a separate procedure (Figs. 38 and 39).

Supratentorial Approaches

Dandy's[32, 33] interest in the pineal began with experimental studies on the effects of pinealectomy in dogs. He perfected this technique so that he was finally able to remove the canine gland without mortality or morbidity. In operating on his first patient with a pineal tumor, he exposed the mass through an infratentorial approach, found the exposure to be inadequate, and in subsequent cases used the supratentorial technique he had developed in the laboratory and was able to report the successful removal of a 4 × 5 cm tuberculoma from the pineal region in his second case.

The operation devised by Dandy is still used in neurosurgical practice and is performed through a parieto-occipital craniotomy, extending to the midline (Figs. 40, 41 and 42). The bridging cortical veins posterior to the Rolandic vein

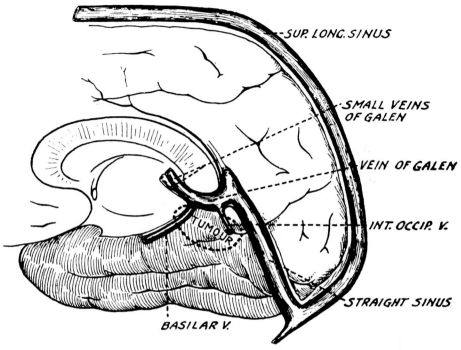

Figure 38 Schematic representation of relationship of a pineal tumor to the deep venous system. (Reproduced by permission from Harris, W., and Cairns, H., Diagnoses and treatment of pineal tumors with report of a case. *Lancet* **1,** 3–9 (1932).)

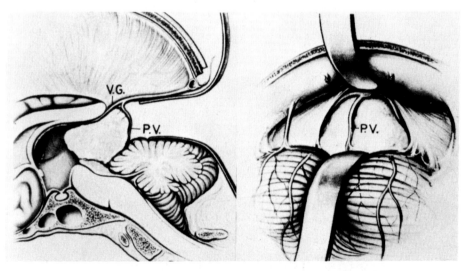

Figure 39 Shows the relationship of pineal tumors to the deep venous system as seen from a supracerebellar-infratentorial approach. (Reproduced by permission from Stein, B. M., The infratentorial-supracerebellar approach to pineal lesions. *J. Neurosurg.* **35,** 197–202 (1971).)

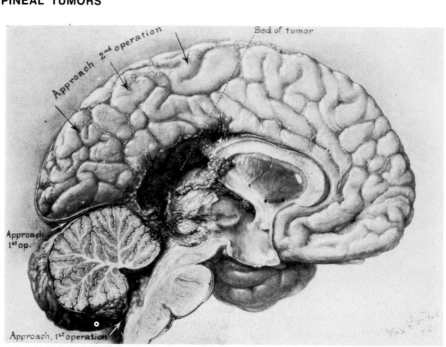

Figures 40, 41 and 42   Dandy's representation of his supratentorial transcallosal approach to pineal region neoplasms. (Reproduced by permission from Dandy, W. E., An operation for the removal of pineal tumors. *Surg. Gynecol. Obstet.* **33,** 115 (1921).)

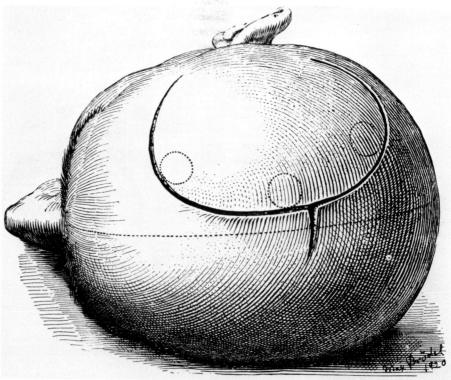

Figure 41

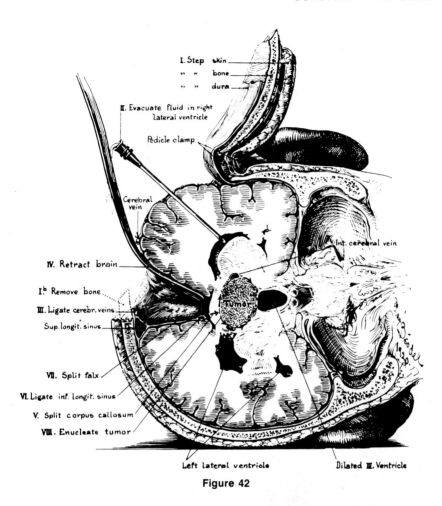

I. Step skin
   „ „ bone
   „ „ dura

II. Evacuate fluid in right
   lateral ventricle

Pedicle clamp

Cerebral vein

Int. cerebral vein

IV. Retract brain

I.^{b} Remove bone

III. Ligate cerebr. veins

Sup. longit. sinus

VII. Split falx

VI. Ligate inf. longit. sinus

V. Split corpus callosum

VIII. Enucleate tumor

Tumor

Left lateral ventricle

Dilated III. Ventricle

Figure 42

are cut and the lateral ventricle tapped to release cerebrospinal fluid. This maneuver allows the posterior half of the hemisphere to be retracted laterally and the corpus callosum to be exposed. An incision into the posterior half of the corpus callosum exposes the deep cerebral veins and the tumor. In this exposure the veins are usually seen to be both dorsal and lateral to the tumor; however, as Dandy[32] described in his third case (and first operative fatality), the veins may pass directly through the tumor. Horrax[14, 19, 33, 34] modified the operation by excising the occipital lobe to remove a large tumor.

The effect of sectioning the splenium of the corpus callosum was minimized by Dandy; however his neurologic counterpart at Johns Hopkins[35] described a resultant disorder of higher cortical function, an alexia without agraphia, in these patients after operation.[38]

Ten years after Dandy's original report Van Wagenen[11] operated on a 34-year-old woman who had previously had a subtemporal decompression and x-ray therapy, and in whom repeat ventriculography 1 year later showed the tumor had increased in size despite treatment. Following a parieto-occipital craniotomy, he performed a corticetomy, extending from the superior parietal lobule to the superior temporal gyrus, and entered the atrium of the dilated lateral ventricle. After the medial wall of the ventricle was opened, a spherical tumor was exposed and found to be adherent to the deep veins at its base (Figs. 43, 44, and 45). It was possible to remove all but a small amount of tumor attached to the veins. Postoperative hemiparesis, hemisensory loss, and homonymous hemianopsia cleared and the patient is described as asymptomatic 15 months later.

Poppen[25] tried the Dandy approach in 1 patient and the Van Wagenen operation in 7 others. His patients either died postoperatively or remained in a permanent vegetative state. Following this sobering experience, he developed an occipital craniectomy, extending to the lateral sinus, through which the pineal region is exposed. Once the dura is opened, the lateral ventricle is cannulated and cerebrospinal fluid removed to facilitate upward retraction of the occipital lobe. A wedge of tentorium is removed and the tumors can then

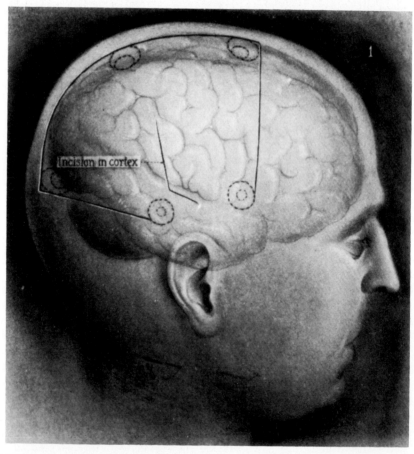

Incision in cortex

Figures 43, 44, and 45   Van Wagenen's transcortical-transventricular approach to pineal region neoplasms. (Reproduced by permission from Van Wagenen, W., A surgical approach for the removal of certain pineal tumors. Report of a case. *Surg. Gynecol. Obstet.* **53**, 215–220 (1931).)

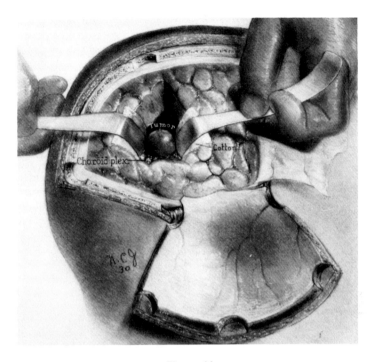

Figure 44

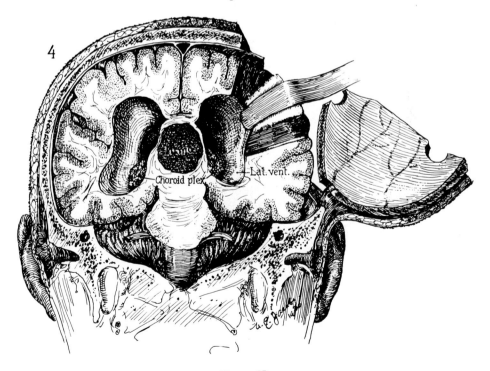

Figure 45

be seen, aspirated, biopsied, or excised. The corpus callosum is not sectioned routinely. Following surgery, a Torkildsen procedure or other shunt may be required if the obstructive hydrocephalus has not been relieved.

A modification of the Poppen operation,[31] widely used at the present time, permits better exposure of the pineal region and less retraction of the occipital lobe (Figs. 46 and 47). In this procedure an osteoplastic occipital craniotomy is performed with the patient in the sitting position, and the occipital pole, posterior third of the sagittal sinus, torcula, and transverse sinus are exposed. The dura is opened and the spinal fluid removed from the right lateral ventricle. The occipital lobe is then displaced superolaterally, with the posterior cerebral artery and the tentorium sectioned from the transverse sinus to its free edge, approximately 1 cm lateral to the straight sinus. The arachnoid of the anterior cistern is torn, exposing the tumor and the vein of Galen and its branches on its surface. If necessary, the splenium is divided. Once the position of these veins, particularly that of the internal occipital, is established the tumor beneath them is removed under magnification.

Stereotactic Approach

Conway in 1973[29] reported an experience with 31 deep-seated intracranial tumors biopsied stereotactically. In 28 of these cases diagnostic specimens were obtained. Six patients in this group had tumors of the posterior third

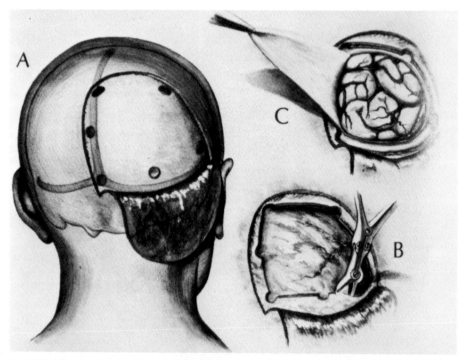

Figures 46 and 47 Right occipital approach to pineal region tumors. (Reproduced by permission from Lazar, M. L., and Clark, K., Direct surgical management of masses in the region of the vein of Galen. *Surg. Neurol.* **2,** 17–21 (1974).)

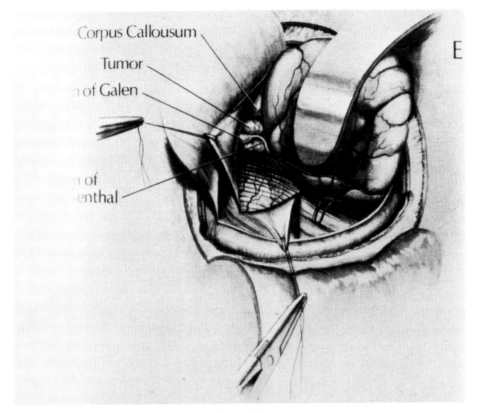

Corpus Callousum

Tumor

of Galen

of

enthal

E

Figure 47

ventricle. Two underwent a second biopsy when evidence of clinical progression was found in the absence of intracranial hypertension, or shunt malfunction 1½ and 3 years, respectively, following irradiation. After the biopsies, which in one case showed residual pinealoma and in the second a fresh blood clot and white matter, were completed, the biopsy needle was replaced by a cryoprobe and the area frozen for 2 minutes at −40°C, 2 minutes at −60°C, and 2 minutes at −80°C. The liquified tissue was aspirated, and brainstem and papillary signs improved. There was no mortality or significant morbidity in the 31 cases. This experience was reaffirmed by Sugita et al.[30] who performed stereotactic biopsies in 10 cases, without complications.

The mortality and morbidity associated with surgery of the pineal region would confirm the impression that primary excision of these lesions at the time they are diagnosed is not warranted. The exception is the tumor that, based on preoperative studies, is probably benign. In the remaining cases, a full and adequate course of radiation combined with a shunt, if required, is associated with the lowest complication rate and the best chance for survival. This impression is supported by several large series, including those reported by Dandy,[14] Olivecrona,[19] Horrax,[15, 20, 33, 34] Rand,[21] Ringeritz,[36] Davidoff,[37] Cummins,[22] Kunicki,[23] Suzuki,[24] and Poppen,[25] in which primary removal was attempted and was associated with a 25% to 70% mortality. All of these authors subsequently advocated a shunt without biopsy as the best way to treat a newly diagnosed patient with a posterior third ventricular tumor.

Since 1971 a mass lesion has been reported as having been successfully removed from the pineal region in 21 cases (Table 9). Although there have been refinements in operative technique, resulting primarily from the use of the operating microscope, and improvements in anesthesia, which have undoubtedly contributed to these successes, I would think that the major factor differentiating the series reported before and after 1970 is related to case selection. Approximately 50% of the 21 cases had benign tumors, including 2 vein of Galen aneurysms, 1 meningioma, 1 pineocytoma, 2 cysts, 2 epidermoids, and 1 teratoma, and another 25% had, prior to excision, been treated by shunting and one or more full courses of radiation.

Stereotactic biopsy needs to be more widely investigated as a diagnostic and therapeutic modality. The preliminary reports are encouraging and suggest that in a heterogenous population with tumors of the pineal region, it is possible to establish the histologic nature of the lesions in a high percentage of cases, with a low complication rate. There are no recent reports of direct open biopsy of a similar population against which to compare the two techniques.

Direct exploration should be reserved for patients with a high probability of possessing benign tumors and for those with progressive symptoms in the presence of a functional shunt, and following a full course of irradiation. In this latter population the options are limited; the dangers of radiation necrosis are substantial following a further course of irradiation and the lesions have a greater chance of being benign than in an otherwise unselected population.

References

1. Howell, C. M. H., Tumors of the pineal body. *Proc. R. Soc. Med.* **3,** 65–78 (1910).
2. Ward, A., and Spurling, R. G., Conservative treatment of third ventricle tumors. *J. Neurosurg.* **5,** 424–430 (1948).
3. Torkildsen, A., Should extirpation be attempted in cases of neoplasm in or near the third ventricle of the brain. *J. Neurosurg.* **5,** 249–275 (1948).
4. Stein, B. M., The infratentorial supracerebellar approach to pineal lesions. *J. Neurosurg.* **35,** 197–202 (1971).
5. Horsley, V., Discussion of paper by CMR Howell on tumors of the pineal body. *Proc. R. Soc. Med.* **3,** 77 (1910).
6. Krause, F., Operative freilegung der vier Hugel, nebst Beobachtungen uber hirndruck und dekompression. 261 *Chir.* **53,** 2812–2819 (1926).
7. Roschach, H., Zue pathologie und operabilitat der tumoren der Zirbeldruse. *Beitr. Klin. Chir.* **83,** 451–474 (1913).
8. Brunner, C., Cited by Roschach (1913).
9. Pussepp, L. *Neurol. Centralbl.* **330,** 560 (1914).
10. Pecker, J., Gilles, G., and Scaran, J. M., Third ventricle tumors including tumors of the septum pellucidum, colloid cysts, and subependymal glomerate astrocytoma, *Handbook of Clinical Neurology.*
11. Van Wagenen, W., A surgical approach for the removal of certain pineal tumors. Report of a case. *Surg. Gynecol. Obstet.* **53,** 215–220 (1931).
12. Sachs, E., Diagnosis and Treatment of Brain Tumors. London, 1931, p. 276.
13. Harris, W., and Cairns, H., Diagnosis and treatment of pineal tumors with report of a case. *Lancet* **1,** 3–9 (1932).

14. Dandy, W. E., Benign Tumors of the Third Ventricle. Charles C Thomas, Springfield, Illinois (1933).
15. Horrax, G., Extirpation of a huge pinealoma from a patient with pubertas praecox: a new operative approach. *Arch. Neurol. Psychiatr.* **37**, 385–397 (1937).
16. Pratt, D. W., and Brooks, E. F., Successful excision of a tumor of the pineal gland. *Can. Med. J.* **39**, 240 (1938).
17. Baggenstoss, A. H., and Love, J. G., Pinealomas. *Arch. Neurol. Psychiatr.* **41**, 1187–1206 (1939).
18. Russell, D. S., The pinealoma: its relationship to teratoma. *J. Pathol. Bacteriol.* **56**, 145–150 (1944).
19. Olivecrona, H., Acoustic tumors. *J. Neurosurg.* **26**, 6–13 (1967).
20. Horrax, G., Treatment of tumors of the pineal body: experience in a series of twenty-two cases. *Arch. Neurol. Psychiatr.* **64**, 227–242 (1950).
21. Rand, R. W., and Lemmen, L. J., Tumors of the posterior portion of the third ventricle. *J. Neurosurg.* **10**, 1–17 (1953).
22. Cummins, F. M., Taveras, J. M., and Schlesinger, E. B., Treatment of gliomas of the third ventricle and pinealomas: with special reference to the value of radiotherapy. *Neurology* **10**, 1031–1036 (1960).
23. Kunicki, A., Operative experience in eight cases of pineal tumor. *J. Neurosurg.* **17**, 815–823 (1960).
24. Suzuki, J., and Iwabuchi, T., Surgical removal of pineal tumors (pinealomas and teratomas): experience in a series of 19 cases. *J. Neurosurg.* **23**, 565–571 (1965).
25. Poppen, J., and Marino, R., Jr., Pinealomas and tumors of the posterior portion of the third ventricle. *J. Neurosurg.* **28**, 356–364 (1968).
26. Jamieson, K. G., Excision of pineal tumors. *J. Neurosurg.* **35**, 550–553 (1971).
27. Kirsch, W. M., Stears, J. C., Radiographic identification and surgical excision of an epidermoid tumor of the pineal gland. *J. Neurosurg.* **33**, 708–713 (1970).
28. de Girolami, U., and Schmidek, H. H., Clinicopathological study of 53 tumors of the pineal region. *J. Neurosurg.* **39**, 455–462 (1973).
29. Conway, L. W., Stereotaxis diagnosis and treatment of intracranial tumors including an initial experience with cryosurgery for pinealomas. *J. Neurosurg.* **38**, 453–460 (1973).
30. Sugita, K., Matsuga, N., and Takaoka, Y., et al., Stereotaxic exploration of para-third ventricle tumors. *Confina. Neurol.* **37**, 156–162 (1975).
31. Lazar, M. L., and Clark, K., Direct surgical management of masses in the region of the vein of Galen. *Surg. Neurol.* **2**, 17–21 (1974).
32. Dandy, W. E., An operation for the removal of pineal tumors. *Surg. Gynecol. Obstet.* **33**, 113–119 (1921).
33. Horrax, G., Daniels, J. T., Conservative treatment of pineal tumors. *Surg. Clin. North Am.* **22**, 649–659 (1942).
34. Dandy, W. E., In Lewis' Practice of Surgery. Edited by W. Walters. W. F. Prior Co., Hagerstown, Maryland (1945).
35. Horrax, G., and Bailey, P., Pineal pathology. Further studies. *Arch. Neurol. Psychiatr.* **19**, 394–414 (1928).
36. Davidoff, L. M., Some considerations of the etiology of pineal tumors. *Bull. NY Acad. Med.* **43**, 537–561 (1967).
37. Ringertz, N., Nordenstam, H., and Flyger, G., Tumors of the pineal region. *J. Neuropathol. Exp. Neurol.* **13**, 540–561 (1954).
38. Geschwind, N., Personal communication (1976).

CHAPTER SIX
Suprasellar Germinomas (Ectopic Pinealomas)

Henry H. Schmidek   Philadelphia, Pennsylvania

A SMALL GROUP OF tumors histologically identical to the pineal germinoma but which arise in the floor of the anterior part of the third ventricle has been identified. Pathologically these tumors have been shown to exist without involving the pineal gland itself and have been designated *ectopic pinealomas*. Since this group of tumors probably does not derive from pineal parenchymal cells, the more accurate term *suprasellar germinoma* is preferable. These tumors represent a distinct pathologic entity.

The suprasellar germinomas are of theoretical interest since their location in the anterior third ventricle requires explanation. Although there are several theories, Russell's,[1] which is the most widely accepted, maintains that these growths arise from germ cells that originate from yolk-sac endoderm, migrate widely in the embryo, and then normally settle in the gonadal ridges of the male and female. Normally the nongonadal germ cells disappear, but when they fail to do so and remain in the retroperitoneum, sacrococcygeal region, mediastinum, cerebral hemispheres, pineal, or suprasellar regions, they form the cellular basis for an histologically identical group of germ-cell tumors seen in these diverse locations. In addition to germinomas, several other types of germ-cell tumor found in the testis and ovary, have also been found in the pineal region. These include benign and malignant teratomas, choriocarcinoma, and endodermal sinus tumors.

The germ-cell origin of these neoplasms is supported by recent findings of chromatin-positive nuclei in a typical pineal teratoma in a patient in whom normal epidermal nuclei were chromatin negative. This finding suggests that the tumor arose from a germ cell that had undergone meiotic division so that each new cell contained either an X or Y chromosome. After a subsequent division, the two haploid cells within an X chromosome reunited to form a cell with female sex chromatin, which differentiated to form the tumor.[2]

Professor and Chairman, Department of Neurosurgery, Hahnemann Medical College and Hospital, Philadelphia, Pennsylvania

Most of the suprasellar germinomas represent anterior extensions from a pineal region germinoma. However there are several reports in which the suprasellar tumor was shown to exist free of pineal involvement. Friedman[3] described such a tumor associated with meningeal and neural metastases without tumor in a pineal region; Kageyama and Belsky[4] reported 16 of 52 cases in which a suprasellar neoplasm existed without involvement of the pineal, and Rubin and Kramer[5] described 8 cases in which the pineal was normal and germinal tumor was present in the hypothalamic region.

Aside from tumors in a suprasellar location, isolated intracranial germinomas have also been reported to arise in other locations, including the cerebral hemispheres, the quadrigeminal plate, and the midbrain beneath the cerebral aqueduct.

Clinical Findings

Even though there have been isolated descriptions of the clinical aspects of the ectopic pinealoma since 1939,[6] these cases were the first categorized as a separate entity by Kageyama and Belsky[4] in 1961. These authors subdivided the cases into three types, depending on whether the tumor represents an extension from a pineal mass, has arisen as an intraventricular neoplasm in the anterior part of the third ventricle, or is located mainly outside the brain and becomes symptomatic due to infiltration of parasellar structures.

Type I suprasellar germinoma is a metastatic tumor that arose in the pineal and subsequently invaded the floor of the third ventricle, hypophysis, and optic pathways. The symptom complex may begin with those typical of a pineal region tumor and are due to acqueductal obstruction, mesencephalic invasion, cerebellar infiltration or compression, and later, hypothalamic involvement. Sequential presentation is unusual, and at the time of diagnosis there is commonly an admixture of signs and symptoms indicating involvement of both suprasellar and posterior third ventricular structures.

Type II germinomas are those that arise within the third ventricle, produce early obstructive hydrocephalus, and later, focal findings representing tumor invasion of the hypothalamus, stalk, and optic pathways.

Type III germinomas originate in the chiasmal region, grow outside the ventricular system at first, and then involve the floor of the third ventricle, the optic chiasm, neurohypophysis, and pituitary stalk. Only late in the disease does the tumor invade the third ventricle and hypothalamus. In cases of type III germinoma, focal neurologic findings, such as optic atrophy, bitemporal hemianopsia, and diabetes insipidus will precede those associated with ventricular obstruction and intracranial hypertension.

Luccarrelli[7] has provided a comprehensive summary of the clinical aspect of suprasellar germinomas, with a review of the literature beginning with the first reported case in 1939. In addition to that 1972 report there have been several additional cases presented in the literature,[8–14] which further support this group of cases as a clinical as well as a pathologic entity. Of the 49 cases available for review and the 2 recent cases of our own, at an onset of symptoms was under 20 years in most, with the oldest patient diagnosed at age 41 and the youngest at 8. There appears to be no sex predominance.

Symptoms

The most common initial symptoms, occurring with almost equal frequency, are visual defects and diabetes insipidus, followed by other evidence of endocrine dysfunction. Elevated intracranial pressure was also recorded, particularly in those tumors arising by extension from pineal region neoplasms.

The visual defects reported in most cases include severe reduction in visual acuity, often in conjunction with optic atrophy, or temporal hemianopsias. There are isolated reports of paralysis of the extraocular nerves and two cases of severe unilateral exophthalmos. These findings are due to infiltration of tumor into the optic nerves, chiasm, and orbit, resulting in primary optic atrophy. As a result papilledema may not be evident, even in the presence of severe obstructive hydrocephalus. Careful visual field studies may demonstrate bitemporal inferior scotomas, indicating a lesion on the dorsum of the chiasm. Macular fiber involvement due to tumor growth into the back part of the top of the chiasm, associated with bitemporal inferior scotomatous defect, is particularly characteristic of this tumor.

Diabetes insipidus is, in several reports, the most common manifestation of these tumors and may, occasionally, precede the development of other findings by several months or years. Hypopituitarism is the third most common finding, often associated with growth arrest in those cases in which the tumor arises before puberty and with hypogonadism or amenorrhea for those arising later. Pathologic obesity, neurogenic hypernatremia, abnormalities in temperature regulation, and excessive somnolence have also been reported.

Diagnostic Procedures

Although plain skull roentgenograms are usually normal, nonspecific signs of chronic intracranial hypertension may be present, with erosion of the posterior clinoid processes and portions of the sella turcica. In an occasional case the sella may be enlarged and eroded (Fig. 48). Enlargement of the optic foramen may also be seen, with tumor infiltration along the optic nerve into the orbit.

Computerized tomography has been abnormal on all cases examined at this institution, and provides immediate information concerning the extent of the lesion and the degree of associated hydrocephalus. However, it is still impossible to differentiate, with a high degree of assurance, the germinoma from other lesions in and around the third ventricle.

Lumbar puncture pressures are usually normal, except in the presence of an obstructive hydrocephalus. This finding is often surprising and may be seen in association with a high degree of obtundation initially attributed to obstructive hydrocephalus but actually representing direct hypothalamic invasion by tumor. In most cases the spinal fluid shows a lymphocytic pleocytosis and in about one-half of the cases spinal fluid protein concentration is normal. There are only isolated reports of the cytologic examination of spinal fluid for malignant cells.[1, 10] It is not possible to estimate the frequency with which malignant cells occur among these tumors, however, whenever

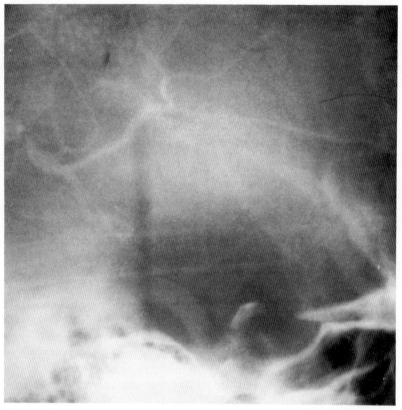

Figure 48 Patient JG, 19-year-old patient with a suprasellar germinoma. Radiographs demonstrate both sella erosion and elevation of the anterior portion of the internal cerebral vein. Stretching of the periependymal veins is a nonspecific effect of hydrocephalus.

the diagnosis of either pineal region tumor or suprasellar germinoma is considered cytologic examination is critical. The germinoma is one of the few tumors in the location of the third ventricle that seeds the cerebrospinal fluid and, if the cells can be identified, diagnosis can be established without surgery. In addition serial examinations of the cerebrospinal fluid, as the patient is followed, may provide important information concerning possible tumor recurrence and whether irradiation to the entire neuraxis may be necessary.

Before computerized tomography became available, *pneumoencephalography* or *ventriculography* was the crucial neurodiagnostic study to outline lesions in and around the third ventricle. At the present time cerebral angiography usually follows computerized tomography to exclude vascular lesions, such as aneurysms or vein of Galen malformations, and also to assess the vascularity of the tumor preoperatively. Characteristic angiographic changes are found in the anteroinferior group of lesions, which includes lateral displacement of the internal carotid artery, elevation of the horizontal portion of the anterior cerebral arteries, and reversal of the curves of the anterior choroidal and posterior communicating arteries. The thalamo-perforating vessels, originally from the posterior communicating artery and tip of the basilar artery, may be posteriorly displaced or fixed and separated. Venous displacements include the local upward movement of the septal and anterior portion of the internal cerebral veins. Larger tumors will displace, laterally, the vein and basal vein of Rosenthal.

Lesions of the midanterior third ventricle elevate the internal cerebral vein and may be associated with other changes due to hydrocephalus. Very large lesions will crowd the thalamo-perforating arteries together and, if the mass is large enough, it will also displace the posterior cerebral arteries and basal vein of Rosenthal inferolaterally.

Pneumoencephalography in the anteroinferior group of tumors will show deformity of the recesses of the anterior portion of the third ventricle. Air in the suprasellar and interpeduncular cisterns will outline the extent of the tumor. It may be difficult to differentiate intra- and extraaxial lesions, since some of these may be exophytic (eg., astrocytomas) and mimic extraaxial lesions.[10]

Lesions in the central portion of the third ventricle may require combined pneumoventriculography because of obstructive hydrocephalus to demonstrate the irregular defect in the floor of the third ventricle.

The suprasellar germinomas, presenting with visual abnormalities, diabetes insipidus, and panhypopituitarism require differentiation from a number of other clinical entities. Included are the intraventricular tumors, such as colloid cysts, choroid plexus papilloma, epidermoids, intraventricular craniopharyngiomas, meningiomas, subependymal gliomas, including ependymomas and the paraventricular lesions, such as sarcoidosis, histiocytosis X, pituitary tumors, craniopharyngioma, optic nerve glioma, nasopharyngeal carcinoma or lymphoma, chordoma, tuberculum meningioma, or metastatic tumors to the parasellar region. Since there are always several diagnostic possibilities in any given case and since neurodiagnostic studies cannot unequivocally differentiate these tumors, biopsy of the suprasellar lesion is essential unless cerebrospinal fluid cytology is positive or it is possible, to biopsy an extraneural metastasis. In marked contrast to lesions of the posterior third ventricle, the intra- and extraaxial tumors of the anterior portion of the third ventricle can be explored safely and carry with them an excellent long-term prognosis. In addition to establishing the tumor type, surgery permits immediate decompression of neural structures such as the optic nerve, chiasm, and hypothalamus, which may be irreversibly damaged during the early phases associated with radiation swelling of tumor tissue.

Surgical Approaches

Several approaches may be used to explore these tumors, depending on whether they are predominantly intra- or extraaxial. For lesions within the third ventricle, either a transfrontal-transcortical approach or a transcallosal approach may be used.

Transfrontal-Transcortical

In the transfrontal-transcortical approach, a right frontal craniotomy is used and an incision is made through the right middle frontal gyrus into the lateral ventricle. The foramen of Monro is identified and tumor tissue is usually seen at this aperture; occasionally a germinoma will extend out of the third ventricle along the walls of the lateral ventricle. At this juncture the lesion may either be biopsied or subtotally removed to provide decompression. In view of the diffuse infiltrative nature of the tumor, should this prove to be a germinoma on frozen section, an attempt at radical removal is both pointless and dangerous, since residual tumor will be destroyed by irradiation.

Transcallosal

The transcallosal approach allows access to both lateral ventricles as well as to the third ventricle. The operation is done in a semisitting position and the flap centered on the coronal suture. The lateral ventricle is tapped and decompressed by the removal of cerebrospinal fluid. The right hemisphere is retracted laterally from the falx. The upper surface of the corpus callosum may then be seen. Under magnification, the pericallosal arteries are identified and protected and the corpus callosum sectioned longitudinally. After the septum is sectioned, the tela choroidea of the third ventricle is reached between the diverging pillars of the fornix. Should the septum remain intact and bulge laterally, one of the lateral ventricles is entered and the third ventricle may then be explored, either through the foramen of Monro or by incising the septum. Biopsy or subtotal removal of the tumor mass may then be undertaken, as described above.

Postoperative Course

Following either of these procedures, most patients recover normal consciousness rapidly, whereas others, particularly those exhibiting alterations of consciousness preoperatively, may manifest prolonged disorders of vigilance after surgery. Autonomic disturbances such as hypothermia, blood pressure instability, disturbances of respiratory rate, and vasomotor instability have also been reported with exploration of the third ventricle. Transient hemiparesis or postoperative seizures may be seen with the transcortical approach and is the main reason why an operation that does not involve cortical incision is favored, such as the transcallosal exposure described above. Ventricular obstruction due to intraventricular bleeding or failure to surgically remove tumor around the aqueduct may also complicate the postoperative course and necessitate temporal ventriculostomy or permanent cerebrospinal fluid diversion by a shunt. Severe memory loss and a Korsakoff-like syndrome may follow surgery and may result from bilateral damage to the columns of the fornix.

Chiasm-Hypothalamic Region

The chiasm-hypothalamic region is usually approached by the standard subfrontal route. A suprasellar germinoma is seen as a reddish meaty structure, often elevating one or both of the optic nerves, which themselves may appear to be thickened.

Table 10.

Table 10. Survival Statistics for Operative and Irradiated Suprasellar Germinomas

Author	Case No.	Sex	Age (yr)	Duration of symptoms (mo)	Treatment	Survival Alive	Survival Dead
Kageyama, Belsky[4]	1	F	13	15	Subtotal and rads	2½ yr	3 yr, 9 mo
Rubin, Kramer[5]	1	F	9	48	Subtotal and rads		5½ yr
	2	M	8	12	Biopsy and rads		1⅓ yr
	5	F	12	6	Biopsy and rads	2½ yr	
Poppen[9]	20	M	12	2	Subtotal and rads	16 yr	
	27	M	19	1	Subtotal and rads		9 mo
Simson[14]	1	F	10	1	Subtotal and rads	18 yr	
	2	M	11	24	Subtotal and rads	7 yr	
	3	F	11	24	Subtotal and rads	4 yr	
	4	M	11	24	Subtotal and rads	5 yr	
	5	M	10	38	Subtotal and rads	5 yr	
	6	F	6	4	Subtotal and rads		5 yr
	7	F	13	84	Subtotal and rads		10 mo
Bradfield[10]	1	F	13	—	Subtotal and rads	3 yr	
	2	F	13	—	Subtotal and rads	17 yr	
Kageyama[8]	1	M	14	18	Biopsy and rads	10 yr	
	3	M	21	11	Subtotal and rads	7 yr	
	4	M	22	12	Subtotal and rads	6 mo	
El-Mahdi[12]	JC	M	19	6	Biopsy and rads	3 mo	
Luccarrelli[7]	1	F	39	14	Biopsy and rads	20 yr	
	2	F	32	30	Subtotal and rads	1⅓ yr	
deGirolami[13]	4 cases				Subtotal and rads	10 yr*	
Schmidek	1	M	19	3	Subbtotal and rads	1 yr	
	2	M	15	14	Subtotal and rads	15 mo	

* Average survival.

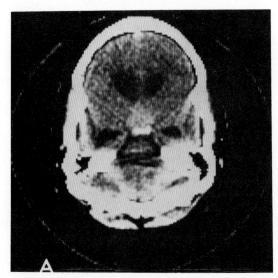

Figure 49   Patient JG. **A.** Computerized transaxial tomography, section through suprasellar region, unenhanced suprasellar mass lesion. Moderate hydrocephalus present. **B.** Same section after enhancement with contrast medium, showing clearer definition of lesion. **C.** After subtotal removal and irradiation. No evidence of residual tumor.

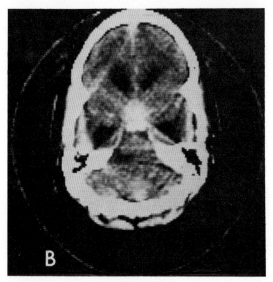

Figure 49B

Results of Surgery

It is possible to glean from the literature of the past 15 years, and from personal experience a total of 29 cases of suprasellar germinoma that have been managed by biopsy or subtotal excision and postoperative irradiation. With improvements in surgical instrumentation and endocrine replacement therapy, these cases would more closely approximate our current manage-

ment expectations than those found in earlier reports. Surgery has been
performed without mortality and with low morbidity. Survival data are
impressive (Table 10) and suggest that in sharp contrast to pineal region
tumors, suprasellar tumors should be explored surgically at the time they are
diagnosed, vital neurologic structures decompressed, and the pathologic nature of the tumor verified prior to radiotherapy. There is little justification for
blind irradiation or suprasellar tumors, without surgery (Figs. 49A, B, and C,
and 50A, B, and C).

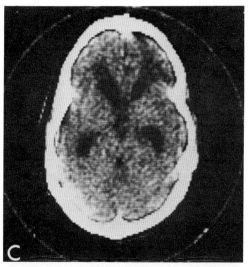

Figure 49C

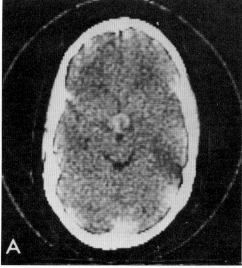

Figure 50   Patient FB, age 15 years. Suprasellar germinoma. **A.** Preoperative computerized
tomographic study. **B.** Same patient. CT scan after biopsy and radiation therapy. Small
amount of residual neoplasm apparent. **C.** After radiation therapy was completed. No evidence of tumor.

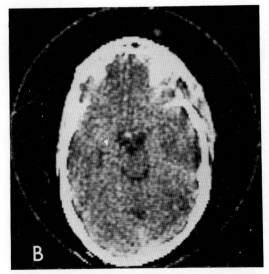

Figure 50B

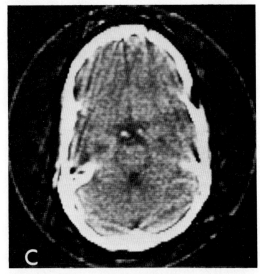

Figure 50C

References

1. Russell, D. S., The Pinealoma: its relationship to teratoma. *J. Pathol. Bacteriol.* **56,** 145–150 (1944).
2. Case records of the Massachusetts General Hospital. *N. Engl. J. Med.* **284,** 1427–1429 (1971).
3. Friedman, N. B., Germinoma of the pineal – Its identity with germinoma (seminoma) of the testis. *Cancer Res.* **74,** 363–368 (1974).
4. Kageyama, H., and Belsky, R., Ectopic pinealoma in the chiasma region. *Neurology* **11,** 318–327 (1961).

5. Rubin, P., and Kramer, S., Ectopic pinealoma: a radiocurable neuroendocrinologic entity. *Radiology* **85,** 512–523 (1965).

6. Akamatu, H., Ein Fall von primarem aus der Hypothalamus-Infundibulum-Gegend. *Gann (Tokyo)* **33,** 371–381 (1939).

7. Luccarrelli, G., Ectopic pinealomas of the optic nerves and chiasm. *Acta Neurochir.* **27,** 205–221 (1972).

8. Kageyama, N., Ectopic pinealoma in the region of the optic chiasm. Report of five cases. *J. Neurosurg.* **35,** 755–759 (1971).

9. Poppen, J. L., and Marino, R., Pinealomas and tumors of the posterior part of the third ventricle. *J. Neurosurg.* **28,** 357–364 (1968).

10. Bradfield, J. S., and Perez, C. A., Pineal tumors and ectopic pinealomas. *Radiology* **103,** 399–406 (1972).

11. Cohen, T., Suprasellar germinomas: diagnostic confusion with optic gliomas. *J. Neurosurg.* **41,** 490–493 (1974).

12. El Mahdi, A. M., Philips, E., and Lott, S., The role of radiation therapy in pinealoma. *Radiology* **103,** 407–412 (1972).

13. deGirolami, U., and Schmidek, H., Clinicopathological study of 53 tumors of the pineal region. *J. Neurosurg.* **39,** 455–462 (1973).

14. Simson, L. R., Lampe, I., and Abell, M.R., Suprasellar germinomas. *Cancer* **22,** 533–544 (1968).

CHAPTER SEVEN
The Role of Radiation Therapy

Luther W. Brady Philadelphia, Pennsylvania

IT IS OFTEN STATED that any course of radiation therapy should be based on histologic verification of the lesion to be irradiated. However, pinealomas are an exception because of the reported mortality associated with the surgical procedure required to establish the diagnosis. Multiple authors indicate that the mortality ranges from 14% to 37%.[1-4]

The primary treatment of pinealomas and of ectopic pinealomas by radiation therapy is generally accepted. With the development of newer surgical techniques, there may be a place for early biopsy and excision of these lesions.

However, at the present time any plan of management requires that the following factors be considered:

1. More than 70% of the tumors in the posterior third ventricle are highly radiosensitive. They should respond to adequate courses of radiation therapy within 3 to 6 months after treatment has been completed, particularly when it is combined with shunting, when indicated.

2. Histologic findings indicate a 35% to 50% mortality with biopsy or surgical removal.

3. Shunting and radiation therapy can be carried out without significant risk in terms of mortality (about 8%) and with a median survival of greater than 4 years after the treatment program is completed.

4. Operative removal should be attempted only in a limited group of patients. These would represent patients with clinical and roentgenographic evidences of continued tumor growth after radiation therapy or in whom a slow-growing, relatively benign lesion is suspected.

The frequency of presenting signs and symptoms are listed in Table 11. Signs and symptoms attributable to increased cranial pressure, such as diplopia, blurred vision, and headache, are relieved by a shunting procedure alone. However, shunting alone produces few long-term survivors.[5] Radiation

Professor of Clinical Oncology, Department of Radiation Therapy and Nuclear Medicine, The Hahnemann Medical College and Hospital, Philadelphia, Pennsylvania.

Table 11.   Pinealomas: Frequency (%) of Presenting Symptoms and Signs

1. Increased intracranial pressure	85
2. Spasticity	35
3. Ataxia	30
4. Parinaud's syndrome	25
5. Cerebellar type nystagmus	25
6. Syncope	20
7. Vertigo	20
8. Cranial N. palsy (other than CN VI, VII)	20
9. Intention tremor	15
10. Scotoma	10
11. Tinnitus	10
12. Other	10

Data taken from Mincer[13] and Smith.[17]

therapy following shunting leads to significant improvement, as determined by relief of other neurologic signs and symptoms and by long-term survival.[6-11] Signs attributable to brainstem or cerebellar involvement are relieved in a high percentage of patients by radiation therapy. Visual abnormalities and brainstem involvement are significantly influenced by radiation therapy, improving after treatment and remaining stable thereafter.

Pinealomas represent tumors originating from the parenchyma of the pineal gland. Zimmerman et al.[12] pointed out that these tumors represent teratomatous neoplasms of congenital origin. They may originate within the pineal body, at the base of the brain in the tuber cinereum, in the chiasmal region, or in the posterior portion of the third ventricle. Other tumors are located in these same regions and represent cysts of the choroid plexus, as well as ependymomas. These tumors may mimic and, in many aspects, resemble pinealomas in their signs, symptoms, and radiographic findings. For this reason biopsy is often recommended to identify cystic lesions that may require surgery or histologic classification of the tumor, since this will influence the program of management to be followed subsequently.

Seeding via the cerebrospinal fluid pathway has been reported in approximately 10% of the patients, although more recent studies indicate that the potential for cerebrospinal fluid seeding may be as high as 50%.[13, 14] In large measure pinealomas or pinealoblastomas are the tumors more commonly associated with cerebrospinal fluid seeding.

Due to the wide variety of possible histologic types, it appears that a dose in the range of 5,000 to 5,500 rads in 5 to 5.5 weeks, using conventional fractionation schemes, is optimal for treatment. In early reports the potential incidence of spinal cord metastatic disease seemed sufficiently low to justify treatment to small fields, sparing as much normal tissue as possible.

At this time appropriate programs of treatment involve irradiating the entire brain to 4,000 rads and then reducing the field to boost the tumor an additional 1,500 rads, bringing the tumor dose to 5,500 rads using conventional fractionation schedules (200 rads tumor-dose minimum, five fractions per week).

Malignant tumors in the midline and posterior part of the third ventricle may be distinguished by the more precise neuroradiologic techniques available at this time. Tumors of the pineal body, colliculate plate, and aqueduct are difficult to distinguish, although data now being accumulated utilizing computed tomography are allowing for a more precise definition and differentiation among those sites. Precise neuroradiologic technique, including computed tomography, now allow for reasonable exclusion of benign tumors and a more precise statement as to the probability of the diagnosis of pinealoma.

With the advent of computed tomography, potentials in treatment have been expanded considerably. It is now possible to differentiate probably benign, sharply circumscribed, apparently well-encapsulated masses from those that are more infiltrative in character. The first type will show no particular change during treatment, so that the program of radiotherapy might be more conservative and the volume irradiated smaller. However, if during the course of treatment a remarkable decrease in the size of the tumor is demonstrated, more aggressive radiotherapy programs should be considered. These tumors are more aggressive and have a high probability of cerebrospinal fluid extension. In these cases irradiation of the entire spinal axis must be considered.

In the absence of surgical intervention for diagnosis, except for shunting, the patient is started on a program of radiotherapy to the entire brain. Repeat computed tomographic scans are taken during the course of treatment, searching for evidence of a reduction in the size of the tumor. A decrease in tumor size during the early part of treatment indicates a more sensitive, but more aggressive type of tumor, often associated with spread by extension into the cerebrospinal fluid pathways. In this instance the program should be extended to include not only the entire brain but also the spinal axis within the volume of treatment. Spinal axis treatment fields should be carried to 3,500 to 4,000 rads, delivered in conventional fractionation schedules (five fractions per week, 200 rads tumor-dose per fraction). If, on the other hand, there is no major demonstrable influence of radiation on tumor size during the early part of treatment, the fields are kept more restricted, delivering 4,000 rads to the entire brain in 4 weeks and 1,500 rads in 1.5 weeks boost to the pineal region, bringing the pineal tumor dose to 5,500 rads in 5.5 weeks in a conventional fractionation schedule. In this instance the cerebrospinal fluid axis is not irradiated, since the tumor is more benign in its behavior.

Detailed analysis of the frequency of presenting signs and symptoms allows for predictions of prognosis and also evaluation of the response to radiation therapy. Visual disturbances represent a frequent initial presenting symptom. Classically there may be paresis of upward gaze (Parinaud's syndrome). This sign is thought to represent destruction in the midbrain tegmentum. Because of this destruction, relief, as a consequence of radiation therapy, should not be expected and most series demonstrate that this is the case. Visual disturbances, such as diplopia, blurred vision, etc., are not uncommon and are mainly improved by decompression. Evidences of brainstem involvement, including cranial nerve paresis and spastic hemiparesis, were frequent presenting signs and were improved in most cases with treatment. The presence of visual disturbances of brainstem involvement is not considered an unfavorable prognostic finding. Evidences of cerebellar dysfunction do not mitigate against definitive radiotherapy and more than 30% will respond favorably to such programs of management. In general, the presence of cerebellar dysfunction unfavorably affects the prognosis. This may be related to the fact that tumors causing such dysfunction generally are larger. Disorders of hypothalamic and neurohypophyseal function may be initial findings. Except for the requirement for exogenous hormonal replacement following irradiation, these findings do not affect prognosis.

Failure to achieve a satisfactory response to radiation therapy may be due to a variety of histologic types appearing in this region. Tumors of the posterior part of the third ventricle may comprise pinealomas, teratomas, gliomas, and cysts. True pinealomas (pineocytoma and pineoblastoma) of pineal parenchymal origin account for about 20% of all tumors of the pineal body. They are stated to have no predilection for sex or age. Teratomas may be typical and include all three germ layers, or atypical, closely resembling seminoma or dysgerminoma. The atypical group comprises the majority of tumors in this region. Its microscopic similarity to radiation-sensitive tumors of the testicle and ovary may account for successful treatment by radiation therapy.

Ray[15] reviewed his experience at the University of Texas, Galveston, with 8 patients seen during the period 1961 to 1975. All were males between the ages of 8 and 44 years, with a median age of 13 years. In 2 of the 8 patients, the pinealoma was confirmed by biopsy, and in the remainder the diagnosis was established clinically and/or radiographically. These patients received doses of 4 to 6,000 rads to the whole brain in 5 to 7 weeks. The spinal cord was not irradiated as part of the primary program. Spinal cord seeding occurred in 4 of the 8 patients 3 to 40 months after the initial radiation therapy program was completed. Two of these 4 patients were again irradiated but all subsequently relapsed. Three are alive, 2 without disease, at 71 months and 43 months, respectively, and 1 with disease at 12 months. Ray concluded that total central nervous system irradiation was a significant and important part of the treatment program and should be done concurrently rather than at the time of recurrence.

Bouchard[16] reported 5 cases diagnosed clinically as pinealoma. Four, treated definitively by radiation therapy techniques without prior histologic diagnosis, are alive more than 6 years after the program was completed. Bouchard suggested that prophylactic irradiation of the cerebral spinal fluid axis would prevent cerebral spinal fluid seeding.

Smith et al.[17] reviewed 20 previously untreated tumors in the region of the pineal body. Fifteen were males and 5 females. The duration of symptoms prior to treatment was 2 weeks to 3 years, with 76% of the patients presenting within 6 months after their symptoms began. Diagnosis was established by encephalography in 1 and by pneumoventriculography in 19. Surgical exploration, but no biopsy or excision, was done in 5. All patients had filling defects in the midline of the posterior part of the third ventricle. The policy was decompression, using ventricular shunting followed by radiation therapy. Of the 20 patients treated, 14 were available for follow-up analysis. Neurologic signs and symptoms improved significantly in 11 after the course of radiation therapy had been completed; the survival rate at 5 or more years was 50%. He felt that these data confirmed the fact that radiation therapy was the primary method of treatment in this disease process.

Mincer et al.[13] reported 12 patients, 2 of whom had biopsy-proved pinealoma and all of whom were irradiated to the entire brain. Eight are alive without disease $3^{1}/_{2}$ to 13 years after treatment; 1 patient developed spinal cord seeding.

Bloom[18] pointed out, from his experience with 175 cases, that the incidence of symptomatic spinal cord disease is 7%. However, it would be unrealistic to recommend radiation to the spinal canal in all patients with pinealomas, based on this incidence. From this experience emerges the concept of identifying tumors that respond to radiation during treatment and of recommending radiation to the spinal axis in patients demonstrating marked radiosensitivity and major tumor reduction during the course of radiotherapy.

Summary

Tumors in the region of the pineal body are rare, occurring in 0.5% to 1% of all intracranial masses. Tumors occur most often in young males. The presumptive diagnosis is made on the basis of clinical and neuroradiologic findings; however, the advent of computed tomography allows for more precise diagnosis as well as for differentiating between cysts and tumors. It also provides an opportunity to evaluate the responsiveness of the tumor to the treatment.

Although treatment has varied from one medical center to another, radiation therapy has usually been an integral part of management. Surgical excision alone is associated with a high mortality rate from the procedure and should not be used routinely. Shunting procedures are most effective in relieving, in a prompt manner, symptoms of increased intracranial pressure. In all instances, however, postoperative radiation therapy should be pursued. Treatment programs for pinealomas should include the entire brain to 4,000 rads delivered in 4 to 5 weeks, boosting the dose to the tumor in the pineal region to 5,500 rads in $5^{1}/_{2}$ to 6 weeks. Evaluation during the course of radiotherapy should be done on a routine basis, using computed tomography, and if radiosensitive tumors are demonstrated, indicating a more aggressive tumor type, the treatment program should be extended to include the spinal cord axis. Radiation doses of 3,500 to 4,000 rads in 5 to 6 weeks should be delivered to the spinal axis volume. Cell-block cytology on the spinal fluid offers another measure to establish the potential probability of spinal epidural seeding.

References

1. Dandy, W. E., Operative experience in cases of pineal tumor. *Arch. Surg.* **33**, 19 (1936).
2. Horrax, G., Treatment of tumors of the pineal body. *Arch. Neurol. Psychiat.* **64**, 227 (1950).
3. Rand, R. W., and Lemmen, L. J., Tumors of the posterior portion of the third ventricle. *J. Neurosurg.* **10**, 1, (1953).

4. Ringertz, N., Nordenstam, H., and Flyger, G., Tumors of the pineal region. *J. Neuro-pathol. Exp. Neurol.* **13,** 540 (1954).
5. Torkildsen, A., Should extirpation be attempted in cases of neoplasms in or near the third ventricle of the brain? *J. Neurosurg.* **5,** 259 (1948).
6. Davidoff, L. M., Some considerations in the therapy of pineal tumors. *Bull. N.Y. Acad. Med.* **43,** 537 (1967).
7. Poppen, J. L., and Marino, R., Pinealomas and tumors of the posterior portion of the third ventricle. *J. Neurosurg.* **28,** 357 (1968).
8. DeGirolami, U., and Schmidek, H., Clinicopathological study of 53 tumors of the pineal region. *J. Neurosurg.* **39,** 455 (1973).
9. Maier, J. G., and DeJong, D., Pineal body tumors. *Am. J. Roentgenol.* **99,** 826 (1967).
10. Cole, H., Tumors in the region of the pineal. *Clin. Radiol.* **22,** 110 (1971).
11. Rubin, P., and Kramer, S., Ectopic pinealoma: a radiocurable neuroendocrinologic entity. *Radiology* **85,** 512 (1965).
12. Zimmerman, H. M., Netsky, M. G., and Davidoff, L. M., Atlas of Tumors of the Nervous System. Lea and Febiger, Philadelphia, 1956, p. 191.
13. Mincer, F., Meltzer, J., and Botstein, C., Pinealoma: a report of twelve irradiated cases. *Cancer* **37,** 2713–2718 (1976).
14. Fowler, F. D., Alexander, E., Jr., and Davis, C. H., Jr., Pinealoma with metastases in the central nervous system: a rationale of treatment. *J. Neurosurg.* **13,** 271 (1956).
15. Ray, P., Olson, M. H., Sarivar, M., Wright, A. E., Wu, J., and Allam, A. A., Pinealoma: analysis of treatment and failure. Proceedings of the American Society of Therapeutic Radiologists. *Int. J. Radiol. Oncol. Biol. Physics.* Suppl **1,** 144 (1976).
16. Bouchard, J., Influence of irradiation on results of treatment of non-gliomatous primary intracranial neoplasms, *Radiation Therapy of Tumors and Diseases of the Nervous System.* Lea and Febiger, Philadelphia, 1966, pp. 153–155.
17. Smith, N. J., El-Mahdi, A. M., and Constable, N. C., Results of irradiation of tumors in the region of the pineal body. *Acta Radiol. Ther. Physics Biol.* **15,** 17–22 (1976).
18. Bloom, H. J. G., Personal communication.

Index